ELECTRICAL INSTRUMENTS
IN HAZARDOUS LOCATIONS

A publication of

INSTRUMENT SOCIETY of AMERICA

ELECTRICAL INSTRUMENTS IN HAZARDOUS LOCATIONS

ERNEST C. MAGISON

Honeywell Inc.
Fort Washington, Pennsylvania

Springer Science+Business Media, LLC

ISBN 978-1-4899-6253-9   ISBN 978-1-4899-6543-1 (eBook)
DOI 10.1007/978-1-4899-6543-1

Library of Congress Catalog Card Number 65-25269

© 1966 Springer Science+Business Media New York
Originally published by Ernest C. Magison in 1966
Softcover reprint of the hardcover 1st edition 1966

Preface

The purpose of this book is to present, in tutorial fashion, historical and technical information needed for an understanding of the requirements for safe, economical use of electrical instruments in hazardous locations. This volume collects and summarizes the most pertinent material required for an understanding of the nature of electrical hazards and the ways in which hazard can be reduced. Most of this material has heretofore been scattered in the technical literature.

The author has not attempted to compile or critically review all material on the subject of electrical safety. This book is not intended to be a sole source document to be used as a substitute for a general familiarity with the source literature; it is intended rather as a starting point for interested individuals who wish to become conversant with the field of electrical safety. It should be emphasized that the reading of a single volume such as this will not turn one overnight into an expert.

This volume contains little new material. Most of the material found here is based on the previously published work of many individuals. As an aid to further study, most of the sources have been cited at the ends of the chapters.

It would be impossible to name all of the individuals who have aided and influenced the preparation of this work. However, the author cannot fail to acknowledge the aid of the following:

Honeywell Inc., Philadelphia Division. Honeywell, my employer, has actively supported ISA Committee 8D-RP12 activities since its first organizational meetings in 1949. The author has been Honeywell's representative on the Committee since 1959. Honeywell has encouraged the preparation of this book and has been of considerable material assistance in proffering the use of both its library facilities and its stenographic services.

Wilmington Section, ISA. The material presented in this volume was first prepared as a training manual for use in the first Short Course in Electrical Safety, held on November 11-13, 1964 in Wilmington, Delaware. The Wilmington Section, ISA, deserves special credit for organizing the course and providing the impetus for the collection of this material in a single volume.

John T. Ward and his committee were particularly helpful in bringing the manuscript to a readable form. The following individuals, moreover, contributed generously of their time and energy in reviewing portions of the manuscript and making suggestions for its improvement: S. P. Axe, Atlantic Refining Company (Chap. 2); L. E. Cuckler, Robertshaw Controls Co. (Chap. 8); W. F. Hickes, The Foxboro Company (Chap. 9); C. F. Kisselstein, Crouse-Hinds Company (Chap. 6); H. Lewis, E. I. DuPont de Nemours and Co. (Chaps. 3 and 4); F. L. Maltby, Drexelbrook Engineering Co. (Chaps. 5 and 10); R. McCarron, Leeds and Northrup Company (Chap. 7); A. H. McKinney, E. I. DuPont de Nemours and Co. (Chaps. 1 and 5); T. W. Moodie, Pillsbury Company (Chap. 11); K. Pinder, E. I. DuPont de Nemours and Co. (Chap. 8); E. Shoub, U. S. Dept. of Interior, Bureau of Mines (Chap. 4).

The author would be remiss if he failed to note the very important contributions of seven women: his wife, Doris, and daughters, Patti, Betti, Bunny, Carol, and Alice, who uncomplainingly let him disappear for hours to work on "the book"; and Miss Patricia Knowles, who typed and retyped the ever-changing manuscript.

Ernest C. Magison

Acknowledgment

Much of this book is based directly and explicitly on the work done by the Instrument Society of America's Recommended Practice Committee 8D-RP12, "Instruments for Hazardous Locations." In other parts of the book the author has freely drawn on concepts, attitudes, and conclusions which have been developed during the deliberations of the Committee. Wherever possible specific sources, such as "Recommended Practices" or papers presented by committee members, have been cited. However, the most important contributions cannot be specifically acknowledged, as they represent patterns of thought, ideas, and concepts developed by the Committee over many years.

The Committee is working in six areas:

1. "Electrical Instruments in Hazardous Atmospheres," RP12.1 (published in 1960).
2. "Intrinsic Safety for Electrical Instruments," RP12.2 (to be published in 1965).
3. "Explosion-Proof Electrical Instruments," RP12.3.
4. "Instrument Purging for Reduction of Hazardous Area Classification," RP12.4 (published in 1960).
5. "Sealing and Immersion Standards for Electrical Instruments," RP12.5.
6. "Wiring Practices for Hazardous Area Instrumentation," RP12.6.

The Committee has led the promotion of knowledge and understanding of the problems of electrical safety in hazardous areas.

Chapter 1

Historical Background and Perspective

GROWTH OF INTEREST IN ELECTRICAL INSTRUMENT SAFETY

Concern of manufacturers and users of instruments for the problems of safety in electrical instrument installations has been, as one might expect, closely related to the number of electrical instruments used in hazardous areas.

In the typical refinery or chemical plant of the 30's and early 40's most instruments were locally mounted mechanical flowmeters, Bourdon-actuated pressure gauges, and galvanometer-actuated mechanical potentiometers and millivoltmeters. When safety was of concern, even the chart drives of these instruments could be hand-wound or air-operated. In such installations there were few, if any, problems of electrical instrument safety. Where required, installation practices for electrical instruments were derived from power and lighting practice; where safety was of concern explosion-proof construction was generally used. Though this might not have been optimum practice, there was no strong motivation either to reduce the cost of such safety measures or to increase the degree of safety which could be achieved at the same cost.

During the 40's instrument systems grew more complex, resulting in very large panel boards and huge control rooms. Small-case pneumatic receivers and field-mounted transmitters were introduced to reduce space and manpower requirements. Safe operation of electrical instruments was still not of major concern even though electronic potentiometers were often used in control rooms. Where there was real concern for safety, the most conservative users still adopted the approach of explosion-proofing parts of the instrument; less conservative people simply used the instrument in its normal operating condition. Because most instru-

1

mentation was pneumatic or mechanical, however, there still was no real incentive to develop a sophisticated concern for electrical safety.

During the 50's, however, the trend toward faster, more versatile control systems continued, with the introduction of small-case electrical control systems. These electrical control systems met growing demands for higher speed and were more compatible with data loggers and computers. Concurrently, an increasing number of quality analyzers were being applied to supplement conventional flow, pressure, temperature, and level control loops. Because most quality-measuring instruments—such as colorimeters, infrared analyzers, chromatographs, pH meters, and conductivity analyzers—yield electrical signals, compatibility of such instruments with conventional control loops biases the system designer toward a completely electrical system. At the present time systems comprising hundreds of electrical instruments in hazardous locations are commonplace.

The change from systems involving very few electrical instruments in hazardous areas little more than a decade ago to systems involving hundreds of electrical devices in hazardous locations forced a reconsideration of the methods used to ensure safety of electrical instrument installations. The cost of previous practices could no longer be ignored when duplicated hundreds of times. The greater number of instruments being used also demanded an increased critical evaluation of safety requirements. Many devices demanded new approaches to safety—many analyzers, for example, are not amenable to explosion-proofing, heretofore the most commonly used method of ensuring safety. With a profusion of devices, the inconvenience and cost posed by obsolescent methods of electrical installation could no longer be rationalized. Furthermore, the high cost of explosion-proof enclosures does not end at installation, but continues as expensive labor-hours mount in time-consuming testing and servicing procedures.

In addition to the economic motivation for safer and more efficient installation and operating practices, there was also a movement toward standardization of safety requirements. Over the years many users had developed their own practices and standards. There were no commonly accepted industry standards of safety. Manufacturers were required to meet individual customer requirements and were not always able to standardize design to achieve manufacturing economies. As the quantity of electrical instruments increased it became more and more necessary to have standard requirements for devices to be used in hazardous locations.

RELATIONSHIP OF UNDERWRITING AND CERTIFYING ORGANIZATIONS TO THE PROBLEM

The National Electrical Code

In the United States most electrical installation practices are based either directly or indirectly on the National Electrical Code. Though states, municipalities, or insurance companies may have their own codes for electrical installation, they are frequently based on National Electrical Code requirements. The National Electrical Code is prepared by the Electrical Code Committee of the National Fire Prevention Association. The regulations in the National Electrical Code are motivated primarily by the desire to reduce underwriting losses, i.e., loss of life and property. The National Electrical Code, therefore, is most concerned with power and lighting in public and private occupancies. Instrument requirements are primarily those for panel board instruments and power control devices, not industrial measuring and control instrumentation.

Underwriters' Laboratories and Factory Mutual Laboratories

The National Electrical Code frequently refers to "approval" by "the code-enforcing authority," who may be a local inspector, an insurance underwriter's representative, or a municipal authority, such as a fire marshal. The "code-enforcing authority" is the person responsible for approving a specific installation. "Approved" is commonly misinterpreted to mean approval by Underwriters' Laboratories or Factory Mutual Laboratories, although in most cases Underwriters' Laboratories or Factory Mutual approval of equipment will in fact result in approval by the local inspector or "code-enforcing authority." Underwriters' Laboratories is sponsored by the National Board of Fire Underwriters. It is a nonprofit corporation for testing in the interest of public safety. Though it is primarily a testing agency, it also publishes standards and lists of approved equipment for the supporting underwriters. Factory Mutual Laboratories is a similar organization supported by a group of mutual insurance companies.

The industrial instrument industry seldom uses Underwriters' Laboratories and Factory Mutual Laboratories test and approval services because approval of such laboratories is limited to specific designs. Because many instruments in a manufacturer's line may be built only on special order, advance approval of an entire line by U.L. or F.M. is not possible. The cost of obtaining approval of even standard items has often proved to be a major impediment to the use of these testing organizations.

Canadian Standards Association and Canadian Electrical Code

In Canada, the Canadian Standards Association Testing Laboratories and the Canadian Electrical Code are analogous to UL and the National Electrical Code in the United States. However, CSA approval is almost essential for use of any electrical instrument in Canada on a broad basis. On-site approval can be obtained in many situations. However, instrument manufacturers generally submit major lines to CSA testing laboratories for approval. The Canadian Electrical Code is similar in content to the NEC. Canadian explosion-proofing practice has followed that of the United States; intrinsic safety practice is likely to follow practices in the United Kingdom.

INFLUENCE OF INSTRUMENT SOCIETY OF AMERICA

ISA Committee 8D-RP12 was established in 1949, in recognition of the fact that both users and manufacturers need Standard Practices to promote safety at reasonable cost. Early progress of the Committee was quite slow. In place of accepted standards of safety there existed a mass of lore, opinion, and prejudice as to the hazards of electrical devices. There was an amazing respect for the letter of the National Electrical Code, but little understanding of its spirit or the underlying principles of safe design and installation practice.

The philosophy of ISA 8D-RP12 has been to use National Electrical Code Article 500 as the starting point for a set of Recommended Practices to promote the safe, economical installation of electrical instruments in hazardous locations. It is not the intention of ISA 8D-RP12 to prepare recommendations which are contrary to the spirit of the National Electrical Code. Its aim is to recommend specific safe and economical practices for those situations commonly found in the instrument industry which are not dealt with in detail in the NEC. The Recommended Practices of RP12 are intended to be as free as possible from arbitrary rules. They are to be based on consideration of the physical factors determining safety, representing reasonable solutions to a problem involving cost and safety considerations, without sacrificing either cost or safety.

ISA 8D-RP12 parent committee has met monthly for a number of years to prepare Recommended Practices for the use of electrical instruments in gas and vapor hazards. A subcommittee, composed of members of the milling industries, meeting in the Midwest, is responsible for preparing Recommended Practices for dust hazards. The work of both the parent committee and subcommittee is submitted to a review board of approximately fifty industry representatives for comment and approval. Throughout its history, but particularly in the last ten years, under the leadership of F.L. Maltby of Drexelbrook Engineering Company, ISA 8D-RP12 has contributed much to the education of the American instrument industry concerning the nature of electrical hazards and the means for reducing them.

The National Electrical Code defined the principle of intrinsic safety in Article 500 of the Code and recognized the safety of slidewire contacts in thermocouple circuits in Article 501 as the result of recommendations from ISA 8D-RP12. As this chapter is being written, provisions in the Code are being considered which will recognize that other types of low-level contacts can be safely used in a Division 2 location. Provisions for use in Division 2 of low-current fuses of the type commonly used in instruments are also being considered.

The educational activities of ISA 8D-RP12 began with the preparation of an extensive bibliography on the subject of Electrical Ignition and Electrical Safety, published in 1959. The Committee has participated in a number of ISA symposia—1954 in Philadelphia, 1958 in Wilmington, 1960 in Wilmington—and held a session on electrical safety at the 1962 AIEE Petroleum Division meeting in Cleveland.

REFERENCES

1. Maltby, F. L., "History of ISA Committee on Hazardous Area Instrumentation," Proceedings of 1960 Symposium on Safety for Electrical Instrumentation in Hazardous Areas, ISA, Pittsburgh.
2. Johnston, J., Jr., "Organization and Operation of the Electrical Code Committee," Proceedings of 1960 Symposium on Safety for Electrical Instrumentation in Hazardous Areas, ISA, Pittsburgh.

Chapter 2

Article 500 of the National Electrical Code

SCOPE AND IMPORTANCE OF ARTICLE 500

Articles 500–503 of the National Electrical Code constitute the fundamental reference document in the United States for installation of electrical equipment in hazardous locations. Article 500 defines the classification of hazardous areas in broad terms in accordance with the nature of the hazard and the degree of hazard. Subsequent articles stipulate specific requirements for equipment, and installation practices to be used in hazardous locations of a particular classification.

Because the National Electrical Code enjoys widespread use and acceptance the provisions of Articles 500-503 have been used as the basis for both API and ISA Recommended Practices.

For those who wish to apply the requirements of the National Electrical Code to instrument applications Articles 500–503 can serve only as a guide to the principles involved. They do not contain specific regulations appropriate to industrial instruments. The emphasis in Articles 500–503, as in the rest of the National Electrical Code, is on power and lighting equipment. The regulations assume a lower average maintenance than instruments receive, and also assume that equipment operates at higher average power levels. Conditions of use are also different. There is little need for frequent user contact with much of the equipment specifically referred to in the National Electrical Code. There is nothing comparable, for example, to chart changing, periodic calibration checks, cleaning, oiling, etc., all of which are necessary in an instrument installation.

Because there are few rules specific to industrial measurement and control instrumentation in the National Electrical Code many users and manufacturers have improvised in an attempt to meet

the intent of the NEC. As one would expect, conflicting interpreta-
tions of the code requirements have often resulted.

AREA CLASSIFICATION

The nature and degree of hazard existing in a particular
location is denoted by specifying the location as being of Class I,
II, or III; Group A, B, C, D, E, F, or G; and Division 1 or 2.

The Class designation denotes the generic nature of the
hazardous material.

Class I locations are those where flammable gases or vapors
may be present in the air in quantities sufficient to
to produce an explosive or ignitable mixture.

Class II locations are those locations where combustible dusts
may be present in sufficient quantity to cause hazard.

Class III locations are those where the hazardous material
consists of easily ignitable fibers or flyings which are
not normally in suspension in the air in quantities to
produce ignitable mixtures.

The Group designation is a more specific subclassification of
the nature of the hazard. The materials in a Group each present
a hazard of the same general character. The Groups recognized
in Article 500 are:

Group A, atmospheres containing acetylene.

Group B, atmospheres containing hydrogen or gases or vapors
of equivalent hazard such as manufactured gas.

Group C, atmospheres containing ethyl ether vapors, ethylene,
or cyclopropane.

Group D, atmospheres containing gasoline, hexane, naphtha,
benzine, butane, propane, alcohol, acetone, benzol,
lacquer solvent vapors, or natural gas.

Group E, atmospheres containing metal dust including aluminum, magnesium, and their commercial alloys, and
other metals of similar hazardous characteristics.

Group F, atmospheres containing carbon black, coal, or coke
dust.

Group G, atmospheres containing flour, starch, or grain dust.

In the United States today there is no recognized method of categorizing new materials in terms of the Hazard Group to which they belong. The materials listed in the National Electrical Code were grouped some years ago on the basis of tests, the results of which are not available to the public because they were made on proprietary items. However, in general, the Group classifications of the National Electrical Code are similar to classification schemes used abroad, which are based either on the ignition temperature of the gas or the maximum safe gap width in an explosion-proof housing with flanges of a stipulated dimension. An NFPA Committee has recently been established to prepare a procedure for classification of presently unclassified materials.

The Division designation defines the probability of hazardous material being present in ignitable concentration.

A Division 1 location is one in which the probability of the atmosphere being hazardous is high by underwriting standards, i.e., where: (a) hazardous concentrations exist continuously, intermittently, or periodically under normal operating conditions; or (b) hazardous concentrations exist frequently because of repair or maintenance operations or leakage of equipment; or (c) breakdown of equipment or process failure might simultaneously release hazardous concentrations of flammable gas or vapors and cause failure of electrical equipment.

A Division 2 location is one which is presumed to be hazardous only in abnormal situations, i.e., as a result of accident, as when process equipment or a container fails. Division 2 locations are: (a) locations where flammable liquids or gases are handled, processed, or used but are normally confined in closed containers or closed systems; (b) areas which are rendered nonhazardous by forced ventilation, which would become hazardous if the ventilating equipment failed; (c) areas adjacent to Division 1 areas where hazardous concentration of vapors or gases could be communicated, unless prevented by positive ventilation with adequate safeguards against ventilation failure.

DETERMINATION OF AREA CLASSIFICATION

Definition of the several classes of hazardous locations in the National Electrical Code serves to establish guidelines. Classification of specific areas is determined by the code-enforcing authority. The code-enforcing authority may be a representative of the insurance underwriters, a municipal inspector, or a member of the corporate safety organization, if the corporation is self-insured. Whoever classifies the location must consider the quantity of hazardous material available at the location, the topography of the site, the construction of the plant or building, and the past history of fire and explosion of both the particular plant and the industry with which it is affiliated. Besides the National Electrical Code, the only available reference on area classification known to the author is API RP-500, a guide for uniform area classification prepared specifically for petroleum refineries. Although the scope of API RP-500 is specifically limited to petroleum refineries, its principles are applicable in any industry. Similar recommended practices for petroleum pipeline installations and petroleum production areas are in preparation.

IMPORTANT CONSIDERATIONS IN AREA CLASSIFICATION

The predisposing factors to a fire or explosion include: (1) the presence of a flammable liquid, vapor, gas, dust, or fiber in ignitable concentration, (2) a source of ignition, and (3) contact of this source with the ignitable material.

When considering the classification of a specific area involving flammable vapors or gases it must be remembered that gases or vapors lighter than air diffuse rapidly. They seldom, therefore, produce hazardous mixtures close to grade at great distance from the source.   Methane gas and light hydrocarbon vapors from volatile flammable liquids, for example, rapidly become diluted in air. Also, liquids of low vapor pressure seldom render an area of any significant size hazardous. Vapors heavier than air such as propane, butane, and many other Group D materials stay close to grade, so that the hazard does not exist long at elevated locations but may exist close to grade for great distances. For example, NEC paragraph 514-2 states that the Division 1 area around a gasoline dispenser extends 18 in. around the dispenser, 4 ft above ground level. The Division 2 area extends 20 ft from the dispenser at a level 18 in. above the ground.

Air currents, the degree of ventilation, and the topography of a location are extremely important in determining its area classification. If there are no walls or obstructions one can safely assume dispersal of the hazardous material in all directions, modified, of course, by the effects of material density. Air currents can seriously modify the conclusions based on considerations of diffusion only: A light breeze can extend a hazardous area for great distances, whereas a heavy breeze will disperse the vapor or gas and eliminate the hazard.

In general, a Division 2 area will always divide a Division 1 area from a nonhazardous area. The only exception is when an impenetrable barrier such as a wall is interposed between the Division 1 area and a nonhazardous area.

GUIDES FROM API RP-500—"API RECOMMENDED PRACTICE
FOR CLASSIFICATION OF AREAS FOR ELECTRICAL
INSTALLATIONS IN PETROLEUM REFINERIES"

Unclassified Areas

Experience has shown that it is not necessary to classify areas (i.e., the areas are nonhazardous) where:

(a) Systems are closed, including only pipes, valves, fittings, flanges, and meters, and the area is well ventilated, i.e., substantially open to the free passage of air. The area may be roofed or closed on one side or may be enclosed with forced ventilation and appropriate safeguards.

(b) The system is closed, i.e., piping without valves, flanges, etc., even if the area is not ventilated.

(c) The area is for storage in containers which meet NFPA and/ or ICC regulations for the material involved.

(d) Permanent ignition sources other than electrical installations are present (this reason for not classifying an area should be used with caution: in some cases the existing apparent source of ignition may be a high-velocity burner so constructed that gases are drawn into the burner and burned at a rate faster than flame can propagate out of the burner. Although the burner itself may be considered a safe piece of apparatus, a match held in the same location might well constitute an effective source of ignition. The relationship between flame velocity and air velocity must be considered in such a case).

It is quite easy to acquire an exaggerated concept of what constitutes a Division 1 location. In actuality most petroleum installations are composed of a multiplicity of Division 1 locations of extremely limited extent. For example, a packing gland leaking one quart per minute ($15–$40 worth of material per day) would not be considered a common occurrence, and yet if a quart per minute were emptied out of doors, the area rendered hazardous would be difficult to locate with a gas detector. Leakage from a heavily frosted light ends pump gland is difficult to sense with a detector only 3 ft away in a freely ventilated area.

Topography and ventilation strongly influence hazard. A gasoline pool in a sizable open manifold pit caused no dangerous readings of a detector beyond 3 or 4 ft from the pit in an 8 to 10 mph breeze. However, a smaller area of a more volatile product blocked on one side produced a detectable hazard in a gentle breeze 100 ft downwind at grade, but vapor was not detectable 18 in. above grade, 30 ft away.

SOME GENERALITIES ABOUT AREA CLASSIFICATION

The following statement can be used as a guide when considering Division classification of a particular area: (1) A location should seldom be classified Division 1 unless it is located below grade or enclosed, i.e., shielded from ventilation, and a source of flammable material exists almost continuously. (2) Except where the flammable material is entirely confined, as in the top of a tank or in a sump, trench, or other depression, an area where a hazard exists more than a small fraction of the time seldom exists outside of process vessels.

SOME SPECIAL CASES OF AREA CLASSIFICATION IN INSTRUMENT SYSTEMS

The foregoing paragraphs have considered some of the factors involved in classifying process areas with respect to hazard. Some instrument installations require specific consideration of the proper classification of the inside of an instrument case, particularly with regard to possible reduction of hazard by purging. The question of the area classification inside an instrument case arises when the instrument case is part of a system which, as installed, provides a means of communication of a hazard from one location to another. Under most circumstances the classification of the inside of an instrument case would be the same as the classification of the area in which it is located. A purging system could be considered a reasonable way to reduce the level of hazard of the instrument case below that of the surrounding atmosphere. However, increased safety, or reduction of hazard, by the use of purging implies that the purging supply pressure inside the case is higher than the pressure tending to drive flammable gas or vapor into the case. Therefore, in all situations where the process material is capable of being transmitted into a case at pressure higher than the pressure of the purging medium, the classification of the inside of the case, even when purging is applied, must be carefully considered. Though this situation is frequently treated in terms of consideration of singly or doubly sealed systems, with or without vents, this author finds it most convenient to consider the problem from the standpoint of a single consideration: if the purging medium is of such a pressure that it is always higher than the pressure forcing flammable material into the case, purging can be considered to be effective in reducing the classification of the inside of the case below that of the surrounding area.

In singly sealed systems, where process pressure is appreciably above atmospheric, this will never be the case. The most common example is a Bourdon-tube or bellows-actuated instrument which is connected by tubing to a process located some distance away, the instrument being located in a well-ventilated area. Process fluid brought into the Bourdon or bellows by the connecting tubing will establish a hazardous atmosphere within the instrument should tubing, bellows, or Bourdon fail. The inside of the instrument case must therefore be considered Division 2 even though the area surrounding the case is classified nonhazardous. No practical purging installation can be arranged. If the purging pressure were always higher than the pressure inside the Bourdon tube, so that the inside of the instrument case would not become hazardous when the Bourdon leaks, the system would not measure well.

If such an instrument were compartmented so that the Bourdon tube was in one compartment vented to the atmosphere, then an adjacent compartment could be considered to be nonhazardous if purged, since although failure of the Bourdon tube would release hazardous vapors to its own compartment, purge pressure would nevertheless prevent communication of the hazardous vapors into the adjacent compartment. This situation is frequently called a doubly sealed installation, i.e., there is one seal between the process fluid and the atmosphere, and a second seal between the compartment to be protected and the area in which a hazardous atmosphere can exist.

A thermocouple in a protecting well presents a similar situation. Such a thermocouple is usually connected to the instrument through conduit. If conduit extended from the connection head to an instrument without any break, then this, too, would be a singly sealed system. Failure of the protecting well could result in the process fluid being communicated directly into the instrument case. Even if insulated cable is used without conduit, failure of the well may result in process fluid being forced back to the instrument through the interstices of the cable. However, if the system is vented at the connection head (the vent may be an open nipple installed in the bottom of the head pointing toward the ground), failure of the well will cause the process fluid to discharge to the atmosphere. If the conduit is sealed in the conventional manner between the vent and the instrument the system can be considered to be doubly sealed and vented. There can be no pressure in excess of purge pressure to force flammable material into the instrument case. Purging can effectively reduce the area classification in the case below that of the surrounding area.

REQUIREMENTS FOR INSTRUMENTS IN HAZARDOUS LOCATIONS

This material is summarized from the National Electrical Code and is presented as valuable background information. However, the material is not presented here as a substitute for study of the specific requirements in the latest edition of the National Electrical Code, which is revised triennially.

Detailed requirements for lighting and power installations in particular area classifications are given in the National Electrical

Code. Interpretation of these requirements for instrument installations is often debatable; however, it is certainly true that Division 2 locations require that, on the whole, equipment and wiring be more stringently safeguarded than in nonhazardous installations, and Division 1 classification requires even more stringent controls on equipment and installation than Division 2. The only exception is intrinsically safe equipment. It is specifically excluded from the requirements of Articles 500–503 because it is incapable of igniting a specific hazardous atmospheric mixture under abnormal or normal conditions.

Class I Locations

In Class I locations most requirements for instruments have been assumed to arise from Section 501–3, Meters, Instruments, and Relays, although this section was originally written in terms of panel meters and power-protective instrumentation. It is, however, the only section which appears to apply to industrial control devices.

In Division 1 locations enclosures must be approved for Class I locations. This requirement has almost always been interpreted as requiring explosion-proof housings. However, the wording of the Code does not preclude the use of purging or some other means of protection.

In Division 2 locations equipment with make-or-break contacts must be provided with enclosures approved for Class I, i.e., suitable for Division 1 location, unless the contacts are immersed in oil or hermetically sealed. If make-or-break contacts are immersed in oil or hermetically sealed, then general-purpose enclosures may be used. At the time of writing of this chapter an amendment to the NEC is being considered which will allow the use of make-or-break contacts in general-purpose enclosures if the amount of energy released by the contacts is insufficient to cause ignition of the specific hazardous atmosphere.

Equipment which does not contain make-or-break contacts, other than the specifically excepted slidewire contacts in potentiometers used with the thermocouples, may be supplied in general-purpose enclosures vented to prevent the accumulation of vapors and limited to surface temperatures less than 80% of the ignition temperature in degrees Centigrade of the gas or vapor being considered.

In hazardous locations wiring must be run either in rigid conduit or mineral insulated cable. In Division 1 areas all junction boxes and fittings must be explosion-proof.

All conduit runs leaving a Division 1 area or conduit runs in a Division 1 area which enter enclosures with arcing contacts or high-temperature surfaces must be sealed with a suitable sealing compound. In Division 2 locations all conduit leading either into Class I enclosures or from a Division 2 area to a nonhazardous area must be sealed.

The above requirements for Class I locations apply to installation of all equipment and wiring except intrinsically safe equipment and wiring. Although Article 725 of the NEC provides less stringent requirements for certain energy-limited, low-power signal and control circuits in nonhazardous locations, the requirements of Article 501 must be met in a Class I hazardous location.

Class II Locations

In Class II locations, i.e., locations which are hazardous because of suspended dust, wiring must usually consist of a rigid conduit or MI cable system, and all enclosures must be dust-tight. There is no necessary relationship between equipment approved for Class I hazards and that approved for Class II hazards. This distinction is covered in greater detail in Chapter 11.

Instrument requirements for dust hazards must also be inferred from those for power and lighting equipment, since no requirements are listed specifically for meters, instruments, and relays. In general, if the hazard is caused by a metal dust specific approval of all equipment must be obtained. If the hazard is caused by organic dusts enclosures must be dust-tight with maximum surface temperature of 165°C, or 120°C maximum for motors, power transformers, etc., which are subject to overload.

In Class III locations the requirements are generally similar to those for Class II. This is to be expected, since the nature of the hazard is similar. The principal distinction between Class II and Class III locations is that in Class III locations the hazardous material is normally not sufficiently fine to be considered to be in air suspension under normal conditions.

REFERENCES

1. 1962 National Electrical Code, N.B.F.U. No. 70.
2. API RP-500, "Classification of Areas for Electrical Installations in Petroleum Refineries," American Petroleum Institute, New York.
3. Simons, C.F.E., W. J. Kögeler, P. C. J. Bijl, "Safety of Electrical Instruments in the Oil Industry," Institution of Electrical Engineers Paper No. 4001 M, November 1962. I. E. E. Conference Report Series No. 3.
4. ISA RP 12.1, "Electrical Instruments in Hazardous Atmospheres," Instrument Society of America, Pittsburgh.

Chapter 3

Explosion Fundamentals

The material on "explosions" in this chapter is intended only to give the reader a "feel" for the development of a combustion wave from a source of electrical ignition and some appreciation of the consequences of changing the properties of the combustible material or the characteristics of the ignition source. The term "explosion" is used in this book to denote any uncontrolled and undesired combustion without concern as to whether it is confined. Our definition of the term includes phenomena others prefer to call flash fires or detonations.

An explosion is not a unique phenomenon. It is only a self-propagating combustion wave which is not kept under control. There is no fundamental difference between an industrial explosion which destroys property and combustion in a domestic gas stove, except that the former is not kept under control. This basic similarity will be obvious to those who have first turned on the gas in the oven and then had difficulty in lighting the match.

Explosions of interest when considering electrical hazards are those which result from a combustion wave on the order of 0.001 in. wide propagating at velocities typically 1 to 10 ft/sec. Detonation waves propagating at several thousand feet per second almost always start as a combustion wave.

During the 1920's and 1930's there was considerable debate as to whether electrical ignition of a gas or vapor is primarily a thermal phenomenon, or whether it is caused by some unique ionic or other electrical process, fundamentally different from ignition by flames or hot bodies. Today chemical and thermal processes of ignition are generally thought to be similar in flame and arc ignition.

In order for an explosion to occur two conditions must be fulfilled simultaneously: (a) there must be a flammable mixture of proper concentration and sufficient volume to support a self-propagating combustion wave; and (b) there must be a source capable of imparting sufficient energy to the flammable material to cause ignition. If these conditions are met simultaneously, ignition will occur.

A complete treatment of ignition phenomena, including consideration of chemical kinetics and thermodynamics, is beyond the scope of this book. However, a detailed treatment is unnecessary for profitable consideration of the relationship of electrical instruments to ignition of flammable gases and vapors. It is possible to view the ignition process in an approximate phenomenological manner and gain useful understanding of it. The material which follows treats the ignition process in a highly oversimplified manner, using simple concepts and models which the author and engineers of his acquaintance have found useful. The material is presented as an aid to visualization of the ignition process. For a consistent, theoretically grounded treatment of ignition and combustion phenomena the reader is referred to the writings of specialists such as Lewis and Von Elbe.

Assume that a point source of energy imparts W_e joules of energy to a combustible mixture so that the local temperature at the site of energy discharge rises far above the ignition temperature of the mixture and a small kernel of the combustible mixture ignites. After ignition, the burning material adds energy to the kernel of gas. At the same time conduction away from the kernel of ignited gas and radiation from the kernel cause loss of energy to the surrounding unburned gas. The gas layer immediately surrounding the initially ignited kernel is in turn raised to its ignition temperature; the ignition of this new layer of gas and thermal expansion of the previously burned gas cause the kernel to grow in size. In the ideal case assumed, it will, of course, grow spherically. The combustion wave can be considered to act very much like the skin of a balloon as it is being inflated. In this case the balloon starts with almost zero initial volume and grows spherically. The combustion wave progresses into the unburned gas leaving behind it burned gas at a higher temperature.

Experimental evidence shows that there is a critical ignition energy W_c which must be injected into any particular flammable mixture to cause the incipient flame sphere to grow indefinitely. Experimental evidence also shows that this amount of energy is related to a critical flame sphere diameter D_q. If the amount of energy W_e which is dissipated initially is less than the critical ignition energy W_c, then the combustion wave will die out before it reaches the critical flame diameter D_q. If the amount of energy imparted to the mixture is equal to or greater than the critical energy W_c, then the combustion wave will continue to grow and will reach the critical flame sphere diameter D_q, and the flame will continue to propagate—in conventional.terms, there is an explosion.

The interrelationship between the critical ignition energy and the critical flame sphere diameter can be viewed in the following manner. This is a gross oversimplification of the conclusions drawn by Lewis and Von Elbe in their detailed theoretical treatment of the ignition process.

In a steady state plane combustion wave (or in a spherical wave of large diameter compared to the width of the reaction zone) the amount of energy per unit volume of wavefront, W_A, added in the reaction zone by combustion is just sufficient to raise the adjacent unburned gas to ignition temperature and supply losses to the burned gases behind the combustion zone. In a spherical wave of small diameter, however, the energy in the reaction zone must be greater than W_A of the plane wave, or the spherical wave will not propagate.

If the total energy in a spherical reaction zone of diameter D is just sufficient to give the energy per unit volume, W_A, required for plane wave propagation, then in an adjacent zone of larger diameter $D + \Delta D$, the energy per unit volume will be too small for propagation. The same total energy is distributed through a larger volume. The energy per unit volume is therefore less. To ensure propagation of the divergent spherical wave, therefore, the total energy must be increased above the minimum required for plane-wave propagation. This additional energy must be supplied by the ignition source.

The critical flame sphere diameter at which propagation reaches essentially plane-wave conditions is determined by the chemical and physical properties of the combustible material. The greater the critical diameter, the larger the amount of energy which must be supplied by the source. Any combustible mixture is therefore characterized by a critical diameter and a critical ignition energy, which are interrelated. The critical ignition energy W_c represents the amount of energy required to make up the deficit between the heat added by combustion and the heat needed to cause the flame to reach the critical diameter D_q.

Another viewpoint, which the author finds helpful when coupled with the previous one, was stated by Litchfield. His view is that if the expanding flame sphere is considered to be an expanding bubble, the ignition energy cannot be less than the mechanical energy pV required to cause the expanding sphere to reach the critical diameter D_q. In support of this thesis he presents the data which have been summarized in Table 3-1.

Figure 3-1 is a plot of similar data taken from Lewis and Von Elbe, and from Calcote, and further demonstrates the relationship between quenching diameter and ignition energy.

The models and concepts presented above represent, of course, severe oversimplifications of very complex chemical and thermodynamic phenomena. However, these concepts provide a basis for understanding the effect of changing parameters in the ignition process.

L.E.L. AND U.E.L.

From a consideration of the spherical model one might conclude that the amount of energy required to cause ignition is so complex

TABLE 3-1

Components — flammable mixture	Quenching distance, cm	pV, mJ	Measured ignition energy, mJ
Acetylene —oxygen	0.018	0.0003	0.0002-0.0004
Acetylene —air	0.064	0.014	0.017 –0.018
Hydrogen —oxygen	0.025	0.0008	0.0012-0.0014
Hydrogen —air	0.064	0.014	0.017 –0.018
Ethylene —oxygen	0.023	0.0006	0.0009-0.001
Ethylene —air	0.122	0.095	0.07 –0.08
Methane —oxygen	0.030	0.0014	0.0027
Methane —air	0.203	0.44	0.3
Nitric oxide — hydrogen	0.635	13.47	8.7
Methane — nitric oxide	0.635	13.47	8.7

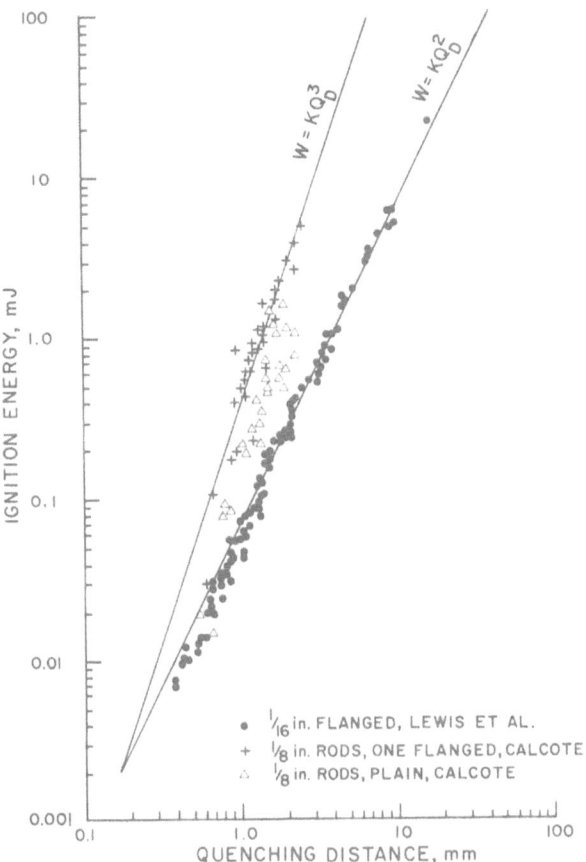

Fig. 3-1. Ignition energy vs. quenching distance (In Calcote data taken as electrode spacing at which ignition energy was twice minimum).

a function of initial temperature and pressure and composition of the flammable mixture as to render very difficult the application of the concept of a critical ignition energy. This reaction is not unjustified. At the extremes of 0 and 100% concentration of a flammable gas in air no combustion can take place; the ignition energy is infinite, and the flame velocity is zero. For the range of mixtures which support combustion, not only is the amount of energy added by combustion different, but the thermal conductivity and thermal capacity of the mixtures are different as well. One might guess that all these effects are related in flame velocity, which is in turn related (in an inverse relationship) to ignition energy. The greater the

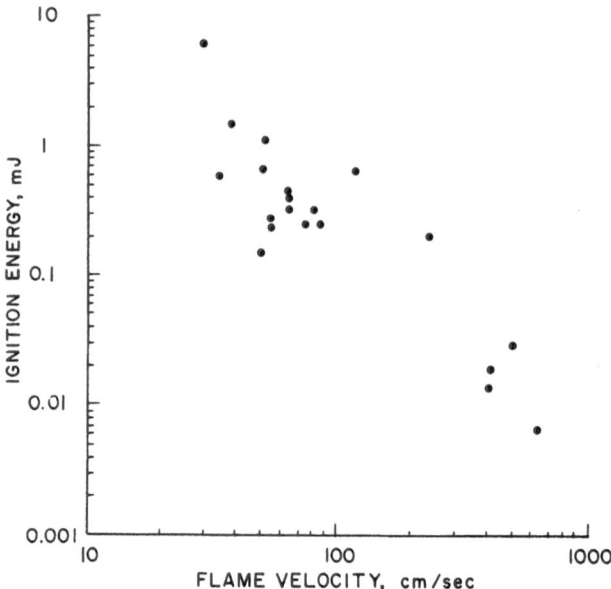

Fig. 3-2. Relationship between ignition energy and flame velocity in 2.5-cm tube. Ignition energy of propane, methane, ethane, and hydrogen from Lewis and Von Elbe. Flame velocity from International Critical Tables.

internal heat generation and the more effective the transfer of heat to unburned gas, the faster a flame can propagate and the smaller is the amount of ignition energy required. There is, in fact, some correlation between flame velocity and ignition energy, as shown in Figure 3-2. Fortunately, however, it is not necessary to speculate in this manner. Although there is no exact analytical expression which relates the qualities of a combustible gas or vapor mixture to ignition energy, no analytical relationship is needed for our purposes. All the properties of the mixture can be experimentally related to ignition energy by considering the variation of the critical ignition energy as a function of mixture composition. If, using a specific ignition source, one determines the critical energy required to ignite various concentrations of the gas-air mixture, curves such as shown in Figure 3-3 are obtained. As concentration changes away from that at which the least amount of energy is required for ignition, the energy required to ignite the mixture increases rapidly, becoming infinite at the two concentrations to which the curves are asymptotic, the lower explosive limit,

L.E.L., and the upper explosive limit, U.E.L. Concentrations below the L.E.L. and above the U.E.L. will not support a combustion wave no matter how much energy is put into the mixture. Burning can occur. If an excess of energy is injected continuously into a mixture below the L.E.L. or above the U.E.L., some of the mixture will burn, but a combustion wave will not propagate from the source and continue to spread.

For the purposes of instrument safety it is usually sufficient to define for a specific flammable gas or vapor the L.E.L., and for a typical ignition mechanism the lowest ignition energy. If the concentration can be maintained below the L.E.L. no hazard exists. If the energy can be kept below the lowest ignition energy, no hazard exists for any mechanism of ignition comparable to that with which the data were obtained.

MOST EASILY IGNITED MIXTURE

The concentration at which the energy curve is minimum is the most easily ignited concentration. This concentration is seldom the stoichiometric concentration, i.e., the concentration at which all material reacts so that there is neither excess fuel nor excess air (or oxygen). Whether the deviation from stoichiometry is to the lean or rich side depends on the chemical structure of the gas or vapor. Most hydrocarbons are most easily ignited on the rich

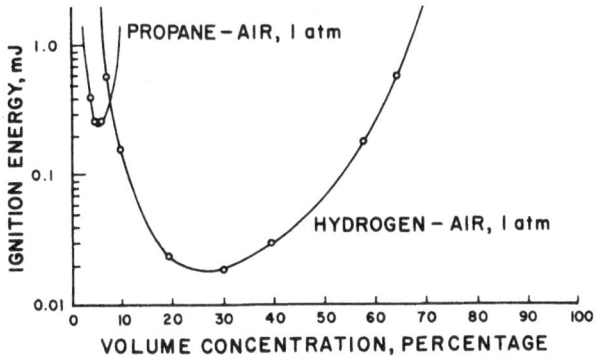

Fig. 3-3. Effect of concentration on ignition energy (data from Lewis and Von Elbe, Table 10).

side. The most easily ignited concentrations of hydrogen, methane, and acetylene are on the lean side.

MINIMUM IGNITION ENERGY

The foregoing discussion has concerned the determination of a critical ignition energy for an undefined set of electrodes. The variation of this critical ignition energy with concentration has been noted. The smallest amount of energy required to ignite the most easily ignited atmospheric concentration of the gas or vapor is the minimum ignition energy W_m. In order to determine the size of this smallest amount of energy, the minimum ignition energy W_m must be measured under carefully controlled conditions. Tests must be so conducted that the most easily ignited mixture is always used. The experimental apparatus must not conduct heat away from the incipient flame sphere, since this would increase the required initial energy input. Much of the ignition energy data to be found in the literature cannot be considered to be minimum ignition energy data, in that it is reported as the ignition energy required for stoichiometric mixtures. In addition, much of the literature data has been obtained with electrode configurations which cause high heat loss from the developing flame ball, thereby yielding ignition energy values much higher than the minimum ignition energy W_m.

The most reliable method of determining minimum ignition energy of a gas or vapor—and the method now used in many laboratories—is the high-voltage capacitive discharge method. This method approaches the ideal in that by using voltages above 10,000 V, the electrodes can be separated by an amount greater than the critical flame ball diameter D_q, which is typically less than $\frac{1}{8}$ in. The mixture is controlled by careful mixing. Equipment is carefully constructed to minimize unmeasurable energy losses from corona or unmeasured stored energy contributions from stray capacitance in the equipment. To determine minimum ignition energy a capacitor of known size is charged to a known voltage and discharged through an arc into the mixture. Either the size of the capacitor or the charging voltage is varied in order to vary the amount of stored energy in the capacitor. Since the capacitor discharges only through the arc in fractions of a microsecond, the energy is assumed to be released in the gas instantaneously and all of the energy from the capacitor is presumed to be dissipated in the arc. Most workers have assumed that all of the energy dissipated in the arc is transferred to the gas. Stored energy is calculated from $\frac{1}{2} CV^2$ and is taken to be the minimum ignition energy for the gas or vapor. A more detailed description of the experimental apparatus is given in Chapter 4.

IGNITION ENERGY AS TEST CONDITIONS ARE CHANGED

Temperature of the Gas or Vapor

In the limit, if the temperature of the gas or vapor mixture were raised to its ignition temperature, no electrical energy would be required to initiate a combustion wave. One would certainly conclude, therefore, that an increase in gas temperature decreases the electrical ignition energy required. This conclusion is supported by recent work with hot electrodes which heated the gas before a spark was passed, thereby reducing the amount of spark energy required for ignition. Figure 3-4 shows the effect of heating a stationary 0.213-mm nickel–chrome electrode on the incendivity of sparks from a moving 38-gauge cold tungsten electrode in an inductive circuit.

The data summarized in Table 3-2 were presented by Fenn. The numbers in parenthesis were inserted by the author; they are

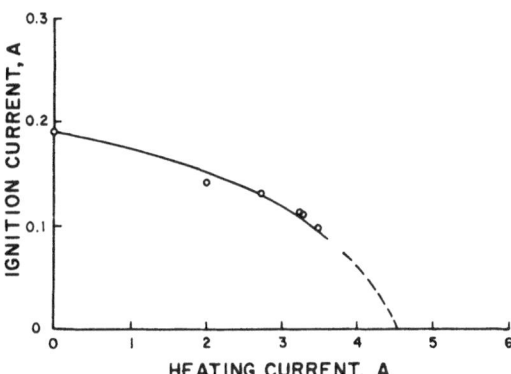

Fig. 3-4. Reduction of ignition energy by hot electrodes (adapted from Rogulski).

TABLE 3-2

Fuel	Temperature, °C	Ignition energy, mJ*
Carbon Disulfide (100°C +)	25	0.076
	100	0.05
n-Heptane (223°C)	25	1.45
	100	0.67
	171	0.32
Iso-Octane (221°C)	25	2.7
	100	1.1
	171	0.48
n-Pentane (309°C)	-30	4.5
	-20	1.45
	25	0.78
	100	0.42
	171	0.23
	175	0.25
Propane (464°C)	-40	1.17
	-30	0.97
	-20	0.84
	25	0.55
	57	0.42
	82	0.36
	100	0.35
	204	0.14
Propylene Oxide (?)	25	0.24
	100	0.15
	182	0.09

*Not minimum ignition energy; mixtures were probably stoichiometric.

ignition temperatures from NFPA No. 325 and are listed for reference only. They cannot be directly compared with the tabulated data since the indicated ignition temperature may be for a different volume of vapor–air mixture or may apply to a different composition.

The ignition data for each fuel show clearly that addition of thermal energy to the mixture by raising its temperature reduces the amount of electrical energy required for ignition.

Gas or Vapor Pressure

When the pressure of a gas or vapor is decreased there are fewer molecules of gas per unit volume. There results a decrease

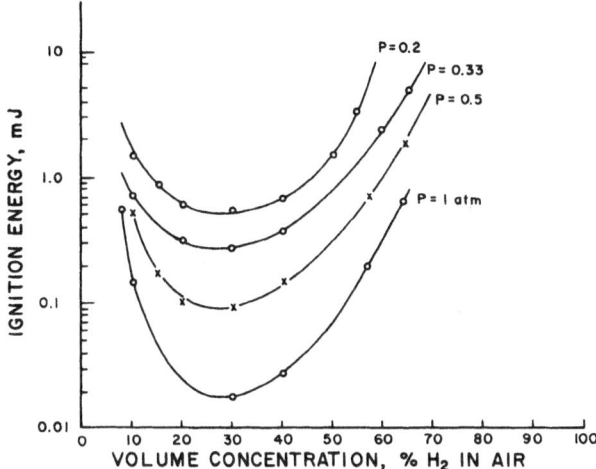

Fig. 3–5. Effect of pressure on ignition energy (data on hydrogen from Table 10, after Lewis and Von Elbe, first edition).

in both the amount of energy released by burning a volume of gas and in the speed of heat transfer by conduction. Both factors imply that more energy is required from an external source, the arc, to cause ignition. This has been verified by test, as shown in Figure 3-5.

Effect of Changing Inert Gases

We have considered atmospheric mixtures in which 79% of the air consists of nitrogen and other inerts which do not take part

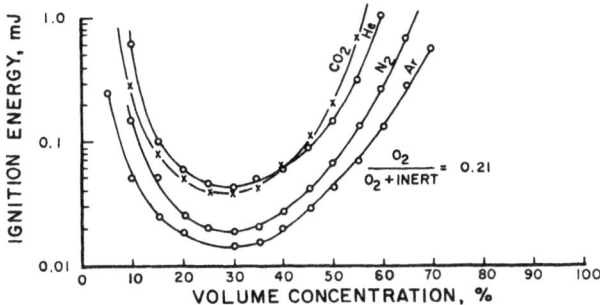

Fig. 3-6. Effect of inert gas on ignition energy (from Lewis and Von Elbe, first edition).

in the combustion reactions. Occasionally it is necessary to predict what would occur if some gas other than nitrogen is used. Certainly, if all or part of the nitrogen in a fuel-rich atmospheric mixture is replaced by additional oxygen, one would expect that a given volume of gas would produce more thermal energy, thereby decreasing the amount of electrical energy required for ignition. In general, this is true. If the atmospheric nitrogen is replaced by another inert gas, however, the effects are more difficult to predict. The data do show the expected result that changing from nitrogen to CO_2, helium, or argon does in fact affect the amount of energy required for ignition. The effect is related to the specific heat of the gases.

Electrode Geometry

In considering electrical ignition thus far we have assumed an energy source which injected a critical amount of energy instantaneously into a small volume of a combustible mixture. We have also assumed that the flame sphere develops unimpeded by electrodes. In most practical situations the energy is not delivered to the combustible mixture in this ideal fashion; rather, the arc which delivers energy to the combustible gas passes between electrodes which are spaced at a distance less than the critical quenching distance D_q. The presence of the electrodes within this critical diameter will result in the conduction of energy away from the combustion zone, thus increasing the amount of loss. The deficit must then be compensated by the release of additional energy into the arc. It will be shown in greater detail in Chapter 4 that any such intrusion of the electrodes into the volume defined by the critical sphere diameter D_q of an unimpeded wave results in a significant increase in the amount of energy required to cause ignition.

REFERENCES

1. Lewis, B., and G. Von Elbe, "Combustion, Flames and Explosions of Gases," 2nd Edition, Chapter V, Academic Press, New York, 1961.
2. Maltby, F. L., "Safety and Electronic Control Systems," ISA Journal, September 1956.
3. "A Review of Electrical Research and Testing with Regard to Flame-Proof Enclosure and Intrinsic Safety of Electrical Apparatus and Circuits," Ministry of Fuel and Power, London, 1943.

4. Litchfield, E. L., "Minimum Ignition-Energy Concept and Its Application to Safety Engineering," RI 5671, U. S. Bureau of Mines.

5. Calcote, Gregory, Barnett, and Gilmer, "Spark Ignition Effect of Molecular Structure," Industrial and Engineering Chemistry, Vol. 44, p. 2656, November 1952.

6. Rogulski, W., "Ignition of Gas Mixtures by Electric Discharges Between a Heated and a Cold Electrode," Nature, Vol. 194, No. 4831, pp. 858-859, June 2, 1962.

7. Bone, W. A., and D. T.A. Townend, "Explosions and Gaseous Explosives," International Critical Tables.

8. Fenn, J. B., "Lean Flammability Limit and Minimum Spark Ignition Energy," Industrial and Engineering Chemistry, Vol 43, No. 11, pp. 2865-2869, December 1951.

9. NFPA No. 325, "Fire-Hazard Properties of Flammable Liquids, Gases, and Volatile Solids," NFPA, Boston.

Ignition of Gases and Vapors
by Electrical Means

INTRODUCTION

Chapter 3 considered the development of an incipient flame ball into a self-propagating combustion wave, assuming that an ideal source injects sufficient energy at the center of the flame sphere.

The development of an ideal spherical combustion wave is a useful concept for study of the effects of changing parameters. Seldom, however, except in artificial laboratory situations, does ignition actually occur in this ideal way. At voltage levels of practical interest, i.e., below 8000 V, the electrode spacing is less than the quenching distance. The electrodes, therefore, conduct heat from the incipient flame sphere. The amount of energy provided initially must be increased to compensate for the additional losses to the electrodes.

It would seem reasonable that the greater the portion of the flame sphere of critical diameter D_q which is intercepted by the electrodes, the higher the required ignition energy. For this reason, as a pair of electrodes are brought closer together the required ignition energy will increse. Likewise, for otherwise identical conditions, electrodes of greater area within the critical flame sphere will require more energy. Lastly, the bulkier electrode, with greatest area within the critical flame sphere, ought to have a steeper slope of ignition energy versus electrode separation.

The effects of changing electrode geometry are shown in Figure 4-1. Although the ignition energies plotted are taken from the work of several investigators who used different vapors and gases of similar minimum ignition energy, the trend of the data

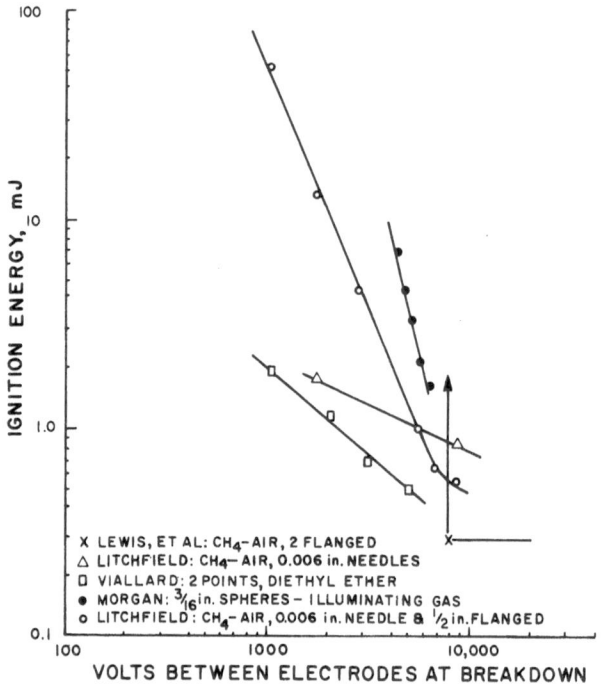

Fig. 4-1. Effect of electrode geometry on ignition energy.

is as expected. The smallest electrodes show the lowest rate of increase of energy as voltage (and, therefore, spacing) is reduced.

At the present time there is no analytical method to relate the geometry of an energy source to the amount of energy actually required to ignite a specific flammable mixture. It is necessary to use empirically determined ignition energies as criteria for considering electrical ignition. Because there is no exact quantitative way to extrapolate data from one set of experimental conditions to another, the use of empirical data requires careful exercise of judgment to determine if the reported ignition energies are applicable to the new situation, and whether, and in what manner, the data should be adjusted.

In discussing electrical ignition it is convenient to categorize the modes of ignition as follows:

(a) Arcing at closing contacts or a breakdown arc between fixed electrodes in a capacitive circuit. In this mode the energy stored in a capacitor is released in an arc as contacts close in the circuit or as the gap between fixed electrodes breaks down.

(b) Opening contacts in inductive circuits. In this mode the energy stored in the inductor is released in an arc as opening contacts interrupt current in the circuit.

(c) Opening or closing contacts in a resistive circuit. Although this mode of ignition can be considered to be the limiting case of mode (a) or (b) as capacitance and inductance approach zero, it is desirable to distinguish it from the other two modes for additional consideration.

(d) Ignition by hot wires or surfaces. This mode of ignition depends upon the heating of fine wires or surfaces to temperatures sufficiently above the ignition temperature of the gas to cause ignition.

Few circuits are composed solely of inductors and resistors, or capacitors and resistors, and few practical circuits consist only of a single series loop. Application of ignition data for simple cases to real circuits is not always straightforward. However, at the present time reliable experimental data are limited almost entirely to ignition energy values for the simple circuits described above. Because ignition experiments are tedious and time consuming, relatively few configurations involving combinations of inductors and capacitors and parallel combinations of resistors and other elements have been carefully investigated. Most investigators, when determining the energy required for ignition by inductive break sparks, assume capacitance in the circuit to be negligible. When testing with closing contacts which cause discharge arcs from capacitors, inductance is assumed to be negligible.

CHARACTERISTICS OF ELECTRIC ARCS

A qualitative understanding of the ignition process can be gained from a knowledge of the characteristics of electric arcs. The first three methods of electrical ignition require transfer of energy from an electric arc to the gaseous mixture. This is not always so in hot-wire ignition, but it is believed to be true when very small wires fuse and strike an arc. The material presented below is intended to provide a basis for a better qualitative understanding of the processes of ignition by electric arcs so that ignition data in the literature can be better interpreted and the effects of changing test conditions can be appreciated.

The minimum breakdown voltage of a gap between electrodes in air depends on gas density, electrode spacing, and electrode geometry. At normal temperature and pressure the minimum breakdown potential between electrodes in air is approximately 300 V at a spacing of $3 \cdot 10^{-4}$ in. These numbers are not absolute; They depend on the shape and surface condition of the electrodes. Breakdown between spheres is at higher voltage than between points. For the type of arc which occurs as a result of breakdown in air between widely spaced electrodes the breakdown process is as follows: if a potential difference is applied between fixed electrodes separated more than $3 \cdot 10^{-4}$ in., electrons in the gap are propelled to the anode, the positive electrode. If the potential between the two electrodes is gradually increased, the current also increases and approaches a saturation current level shown as point A in Figure 4-2. At some critical value of applied potential the current will increase rapidly. This is the characteristic breakdown of the gap, section B of the curve in Figure 4-2.

During the initial application to the gap of voltages below the breakdown voltage, electrons drawn to the anode are those which were initially present in the gap. Some electrons are always present, usually from collision of gamma rays with gas molecules,

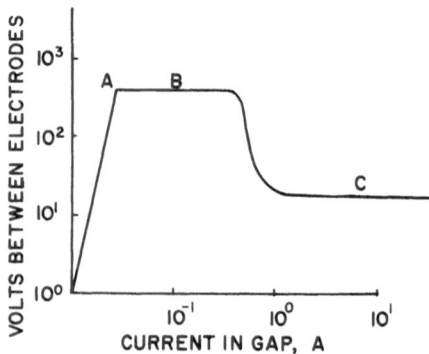

Fig. 4-2. Gap voltage–current curve before and after breakdown.

or by photon action on the electrode material. Many electrons cannot complete the journey from cathode to anode because they collide with gas molecules along the way and drift back to the cathode, or are forced back by space charge. As the potential between electrodes is increased more electrons are given a velocity component in the direction of the anode and survive successive collisions with molecules of gas to reach the anode. At the saturation current level the number of electrons reaching the anode is primarily dependent upon the number of electrons initially in the gap. As the potential between the electrodes is raised, some electrons gain sufficient energy so that they displace an additional electron from a gas molecule by collision, increasing the total number of electrons available to cross the gap. At the critical potential, called the breakdown voltage, the field strength is so high that collision-produced electrons outnumber those lost by collision and an "avalanche" occurs; i.e., when, on the average, each electron produces additional electrons by collision, so that the number of electrons in the gap increases exponentially, breakdown is said to have occurred. After breakdown, if the current is limited to values on the order of 0.1 A, the voltage across the electrodes generally remains at about the level of minimum breakdown voltage in air, about 300 V, and the discharge is called a glow discharge. The exact voltage is a function of the materials of the anode and cathode, the spacing of the electrodes, and the current. Increasing the current causes a transition from the glow discharge to a low-voltage arc discharge as shown in region C of Figure 4-2. The voltage between electrodes drops to a lower value. The characteristics of the low-voltage arc discharge will be further described below.

Because the breakdown of the gap between electrodes depends upon enough electrons acquiring sufficient energy to displace additional electrons from molecules of gas, breakdown does not occur immediately upon application of the minimum breakdown voltage. Although free electrons caused by cosmic radiation are always present, they may be so few in number that a significant amount of time can elapse before a naturally produced electron is in such a favorable position in the gap that application of the minimum breakdown voltage will result in avalanche breakdown. Therefore, it is often necessary to apply a voltage greater than the normal minimum breakdown voltage in order to induce breakdown. For this reason, in ignition testing the possibility of abnormally high breakdown voltage is usually eliminated by irradiating the gap with an ultraviolet source, a radioactive source, or a small auxiliary arc which produces ultraviolet radiation, to ensure an ample initial supply of electrons.

Since much electrical equipment contains no voltages even as high as the 300 V minimum sparking potential in air, the characteristics of the low-voltage arc are of greater pertinence to the study of electrical ignition than those of the glow discharge. Because 300 V is the minimum sparking potential in air at normal temperature and pressure, one might conclude that discharge arcs are not possible below this potential. However, anyone who has accidentally touched a screwdriver to a 12 V automobile battery knows that sizable (not necessarily ignition-capable) arcs can be generated at these low voltages with a purely resistive load. It is certainly not necessary to obtain a glow discharge at first.

Controversy still exists as to the initiating mechanism of low-voltage arcs between electrodes which are slowly brought together. One point of view holds that electrostatic fields of the order of 10^7 V/in. are sufficient to extract electrons even from cold metals, and that microscopic surface irregularities reduce the required applied potential to a value equivalent to 10^6 V/in. in terms of gross electrode spacing. A second point of view is that when two contacts are brought together current first flows when ohmic contact is made by a whisker of metal or carbon. Current then vaporizes the whisker and provides conducting vapor to start an arc. It is not of particular concern in ignition work which theory more closely describes the actual physical processes. The breakdown data obtained by investigators who hold to both views gives essentially the same sort of information, i.e., that the breakdown voltage gradient below the minimum sparking potential in air is approximately 10^6 V/in. Figure 4-3 illustrates the relationship between contact separation and breakdown voltage.

Whether a short arc is formed by opening a current-carrying circuit, by closing a circuit lower than the sparking potential and causing an arc, or by breakdown between two electrodes at voltage above the minimum sparking potential in air and then drawing enough current to cause transition from a glow discharge to an arc discharge, the characteristics of the final arc are the same in the steady state.

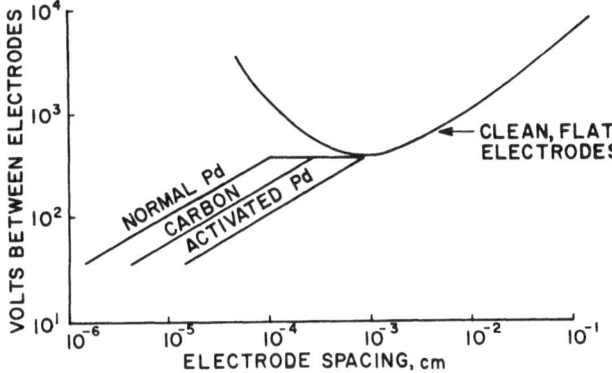

Fig. 4-3. Breakdown voltage between electrodes in air.

The characteristics of a stable arc can most effectively be described by a family of voltage–current curves with electrode spacing as a parameter. Sets of curves for tungsten and carbon electrodes are shown in Figure 4-4. Curves for other materials are similar, but the minimum current I_m and the minimum voltage V_m, to which the limiting (0 mm) curves are asymptotic, change with changes in the material. Table 4-1 gives values for some metals for arcs in air, in nitrogen, and in hydrogen; the values are taken

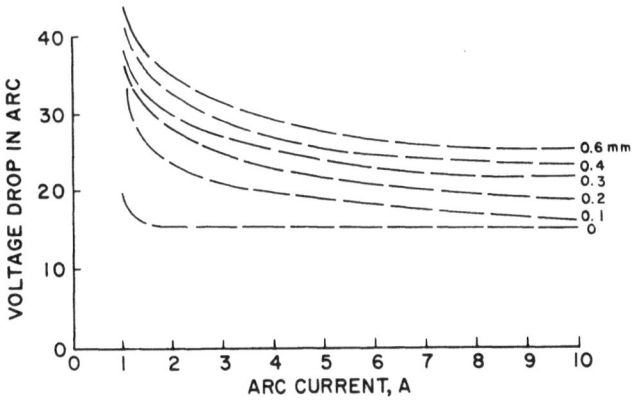

Fig. 4-4a. Arc characteristics—tungsten (from Holm, Fig. 53.05).

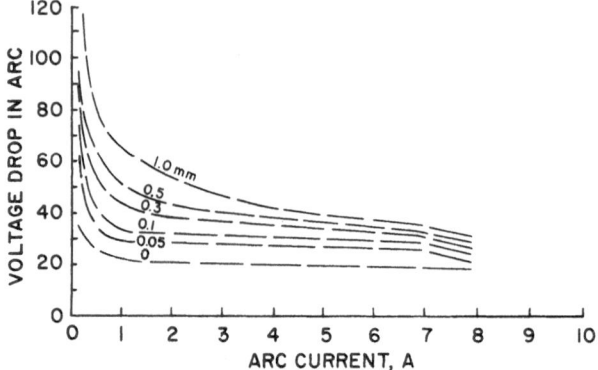

Fig. 4-4b. Arc characteristics—carbon (from Holm, Fig. 53.04).

TABLE 4-1

Minimum Voltage and Current Values for
Stable Arcs for Various Metals

Material	V_m, V	I_m, A
Carbon	20	0.03
Aluminum	14	—
Iron	13 — 15	0.35 — 0.55
Nickel	14	0.5
Copper in nitrogen	14	0.6
Copper in air	13	0.43
Copper in hydrogen	18	1.3
Silver in air	12	0.4
Silver in nitrogen	13	0.8
Silver in hydrogen	21	—
Cadmium in nitrogen	11	0.1
Tin	13.5	—
Gold in air	15	0.38
Gold in hydrogen	20	—
Tungsten	15	1
Platinum	17.5	0.9
Stainless steel	15	0.5

from Holm. The V_m and I_m values reported by other investigators may differ by 20–30%.

It is of interest to note that carbon arcs can be stable at very low current levels, far lower than any other material listed. It is likely that in many practical situations arcing of metallic contacts is at voltage and current levels near those typical of carbon electrodes, either because of carbonaceous dirt or because of contamination by surrounding hydrocarbon atmospheres. The latter effect is notable in affecting the breakdown voltage, as shown in Figure 4-3. The normal palladium electrode (one which is clean) requires higher voltage at given separation than a carbon electrode. A palladium electrode "activated" by arcing in certain hydrocarbon vapors requires still lower voltage to cause breakdown. These effects provide an explanation, though not the only one, for ignition in resistive circuits at circuit voltage and initial current which is incompatible with the arc characteristics of the electrode material. Ignition when breaking a 125 V resistive circuit at 0.9 A with platinum electrodes has been reported. The values for platinum in Table 4-1 are 17.5 V and 0.9 A as asymptotes. A load line drawn from 125 V to 0.9 A initial current would not cross a point on the arc characteristic. For an electrode modified by a carbon deposit such a load line would be possible.

ARCING AT CLOSING CONTACTS AND IN CAPACITIVE CIRCUITS

Capacitive discharge arcs have been studied by investigators with two quite different interests. The method of igniting gases with discharge arcs from small capacitors charged to high voltage was brought to a high state of sophistication at the U.S. Bureau of Mines in Pittsburgh, where it was used to measure the minimum ignition energy of gases, vapors, and dusts. These investigators were interested in determining minimum ignition energy of gases and vapors first for application to ignition and combustion theory and secondly for application to problems of safety. Their principal interest, however, was in the determination of an absolute minimum ignition energy for use in theories of combustion and ignition.

In these investigations the potentials were sufficiently high that electrode spacing was greater than the quenching distance of the gas or vapor being tested. Therefore, thermal losses from the

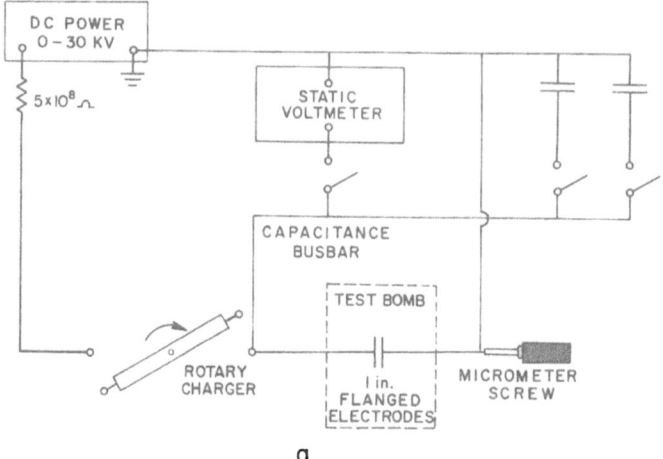

a

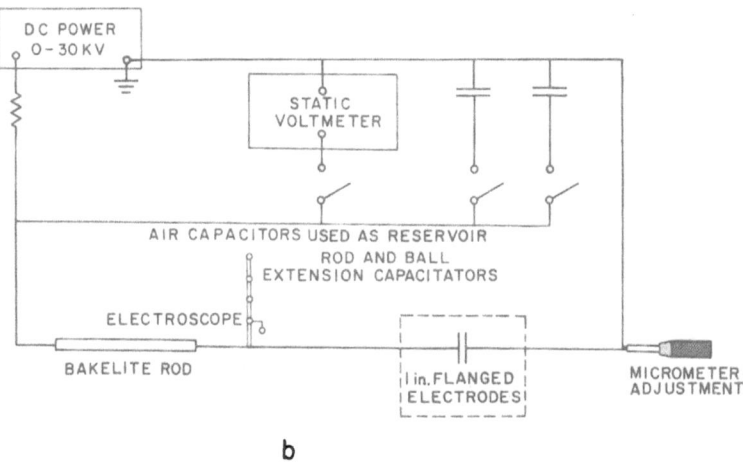

b

Fig. 4-5. Bureau of Mines high-voltage test apparatus; a) apparatus for capacitance greater than 100 pF; b) apparatus for capacitance less than 100 pF.

spark, except to the surrounding gas, were very small. Because electrode spacing was greater than the quenching distance, when the expanding gas sphere reached the electrodes it was already bigger than the critical diameter D_q, and was self-sustaining. Removal of energy from the combustion wave by the electrodes therefore did not require additional energy to initiate the explosion. Because there are only small thermal losses from the spark (except to the surrounding gas) it is assumed in such high-voltage minimum ignition energy determinations that all of the energy stored in the capacitor is discharged in the arc and absorbed by the gas. The total energy delivered to the gas is the energy stored on the capacitor, $\frac{1}{2} CV^2$, where C is the value of the capacitor in farads and V is the voltage to which the capacitor is charged.

The high-voltage discharge test equipment used by Blanc, Guest, Von Elbe, and Lewis was of two types (see Figure 4-5). For relatively large capacitors, those larger than $100 \, \mu\mu$ F, a DC voltage supply was used. The test capacitor, connected to electrodes mounted within a test bomb, was slowly charged by a rotating charging rod which transferred charge from the DC power supply to the test capacitor. A test capacitor size was selected and the spacing between electrodes was adjusted for a given test series. The voltage on the test capacitor was then slowly increased by rotating the charging rod until breakdown occurred. In order to remove uncertainties in data due to the statistical time lag of breakdown, the gap was irradiated by a radium source.

When testing capacitors smaller than $100 \, \mu\mu$ F the rotary charger was replaced by a Bakelite rod connected continuously to the test capacitor. The grounded electrode was then moved to reduce the gap distance to cause breakdown. In both cases the apparatus was very carefully constructed to minimize the amount of stray capacitance in leads, to eliminate any contribution of energy by continuous steady state current from the source, and to minimize any bias on data caused by inductance and resistance in the electrode circuits. The electrodes used in obtaining data were pointed or flanged. Typical ignition energy versus electrode separation plots

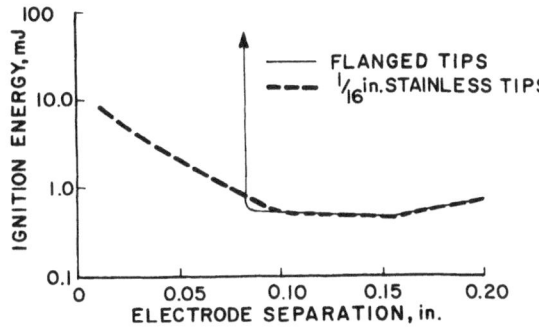

Fig. 4-6. Ignition energy vs. distance (adapted from Lewis and Von Elbe).

are shown in Figure 4-6. Note that when flanged electrodes are used there is an appreciable range of spacings just greater than the quenching distance over which the ignition energy is relatively constant. However, the amount of energy required to cause ignition at the quenching distance increases at an almost infinite rate. If the flanged electrodes are replaced by pointed electrodes the amount of energy required for ignition begins to increase near the quenching distance, but at a rate which is now dependent upon electrode geometry, as was shown in Figure 4-1. It was on the basis of such experimental data as these that the concept of a minimum flame ball diameter was developed. If flanged electrodes are used at spacings below the quenching distance and the arc is confined to the center of the flange, even though a large amount of energy is dissipated between the flanges, the flame sphere cannot grow to the critical diameter where the rate of heat generated by combustion equals or exceeeds the rate of heat lost through the surroundings. The flanged electrodes conduct large amounts of heat away from the flame zone. Pointed electrodes also conduct heat away from the combustion zone, but, because they are relatively much smaller than flanged electrodes, the rate of increase of energy required to offset the conductive effects of the electrodes as they are brought closer together is much smaller. The Bureau of Mines investigators found that for best control it was necessary to use glass flanges on the electrodes in order to confine the arc always to the center of the flange. They found similar quenching effects with either glass or metal flanges, since the ratio of the thermal conductivity of a solid to that of a gas is so large that differences between solids are immaterial. Glass flanges are recommended because metal flanges, being electrically conductive, will occasionally support an arc at the edge of the flange, causing ignition even when the flanges are within the quenching distance.

Figure 4-6 shows also that as the distance between electrodes increases the amount of energy required for ignition eventually begins to increase. This can be explained qualitatively on the basis of the fact that as the length of the arc is increased the amount of energy required to support the arc must be increased. Photographs of ignition by such long arcs have shown that instead of a single incipient flame sphere developing from the arc, several incipient flame balls may develop, requiring the expenditure of more than the minimum ignition energy.

The results of the Bureau of Mines investigations have contributed substantially to the understanding of the ignition mechanism.
The method is extremely important in obtaining an absolute measure
of minimum ignition energy, so that the ignitibilities of gases and
vapors can be effectively compared. The energies measured in
such high-voltage ignition tests are not, however, directly applicable
to problems of electrical safety, especially those which are common
in the instrument industry. The voltages used in these tests are
impractically high. In addition, all the conditions in this type of
testing are controlled to eliminate energy loss. Such conditions
are not attained in practical instrument systems. High-voltage
ignition data may, of course, be specifically and directly pertinent
in ignition by static discharges.

Most instrument systems operate well below 1000 V, but
breakdown at even 1000 V corresponds to approximately 0.005-in.
electrode separation in air. The quenching distance for most
materials is in the range 0.02 in.–0.12 in. Quenching by the electrodes in practical ignition mechanisms is therefore important at
any operating voltage. Quenching becomes even more important in
arcs at lower voltages which can be initiated only at spacings on
the order of tens and hundreds of microinches. Because electrodes
are inside the flame sphere it is very difficult to obtain reproducible
data on ignition energy for low-voltage conditions. Comparison of
data from different investigators is also difficult. The specific
geometry and materials of the electrodes determine test results.
Because the electrode spacing at low voltages is of the order of
10^{-5} in., changes in surface geometry invisible to the naked eye
may have large effects on the amount of energy required to cause
ignition.

TYPICAL TEST EQUIPMENT FOR CAPACITIVE CIRCUITS

In the United Kingdom the ignition capability of capacitive discharge sparks has been determined using the "intermittent break
apparatus." In this apparatus the circuit is broken between two
pieces of platinum alloy strip 0.009 in. (0.23 mm) in thickness. The
edge of one of these strips, which is 0.2 in. wide, is cut to form a
sawtooth with eleven teeth. This is drawn across the straight edge
of the other strip to produce a succession of ten sparks at each
operation. These electrodes are operated in the "break-flash"

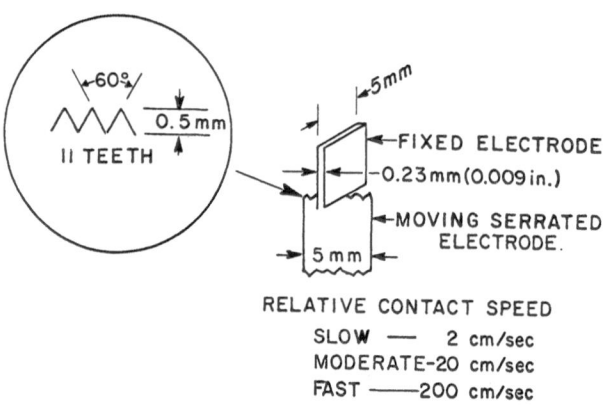

Fig. 4-7. "Intermittent break" apparatus electrodes.

apparatus (to be described later under "Inductive Break-Spark Testing"), such that the ten sparks take place in about 0.21 sec. The interval between successive sparks is therefore about 0.02 sec. Figure 4-7 shows the main features of this method. Curve F in Figure 4-10a represents data from similar apparatus in France.

Allsop and Guénault reported results obtained by manually closing electrodes in Safety in Mines Research Paper No. 107. Data for a platinum point and rod are shown as Curve E_1 in Figure 4-10a.

Curve E in Figure 4-10a represents ignition caused by discharge of capacitors through 0.015-in. lengths of 0.0005-in. nichrome wire. Fusing of the wire causes an arc. This apparatus is not used for routine testing, but was constructed at the Safety in Mines Research Establishment because it has the advantage of using a fresh electrode pair for each test.

In Germany, at the Physikalisch-Technische Bundesanstalt (PTB), a counter-rotating brush and a slotted disc, as shown in Figure 4-8, are used for testing the ignition capability of all kinds of sparks. Suspended from one disc are four tungsten wires of 0.008 in. (0.2 mm) diameter. The wires are 0.44 in. (11 mm) long. A cadmium disc is mounted so that its top surface is 0.4 in. below the rotating tungsten wire holder. The cadmium disc has machined in it two chordal grooves 0.080 in. wide by 0.080 in. deep. The tungsten wire contact holder revolves at 90 rpm; the cadmium disc rotates in the opposite direction at approximately 20 rpm. As can be seen from the figure, the counter-rotating discs cause the tungsten wire to approach the edge of the disc, scrape across the surface of the cadmium disc, and bend the wire, thereby providing a relatively fast break as the wire springs on the edge of the slot. A slow make will occur as the wire comes against the side of the slot; a slow break, as the wire and slot move relative to one another; and a relatively fast break, as the wire and disc break contact for the last time in the cycle. It is the author's understanding that steel wire is used in place of tungsten for routine tests, in which case ignition levels are not significantly different. The steel wire has longer life than tungsten wire, which breaks frequently.

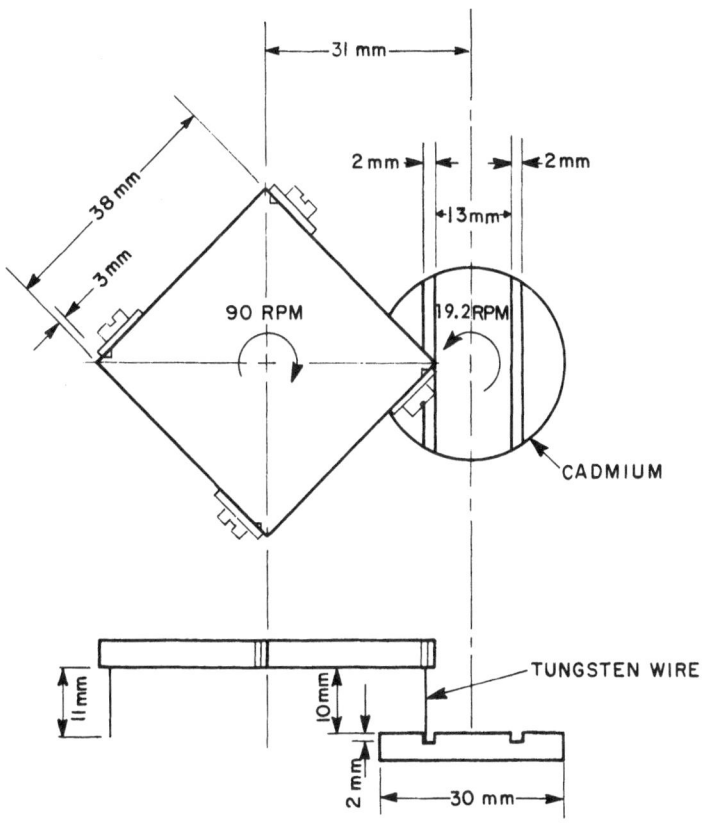

Fig. 4-8. PTB test apparatus.

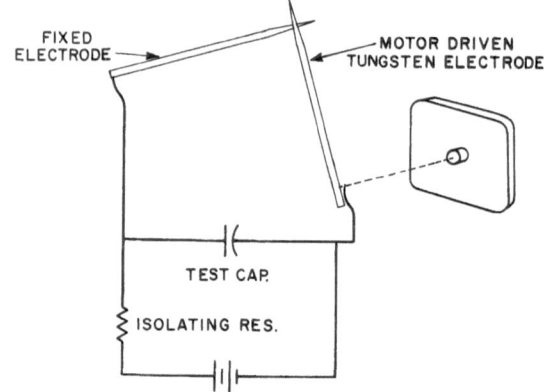

FIXED
ELECTRODE

MOTOR DRIVEN
TUNGSTEN ELECTRODE

TEST CAP.

ISOLATING RES.

ELECTRODES: 0.025 in. TUNGSTEN WIRE, DRAWN TO POINT
CONTACTING AT 0.005 in. DIA.

Fig. 4-9. Magison's test apparatus.

In his own investigations the author used 0.025 in. diameter tungsten wire sharpened at the end. One wire was held stationary while the second wire was rotated at right angles to the first, so that contact was made at a speed of approximately 0.1 in./sec. (see Figure 4-9).

PRECAUTIONS IN TESTING

Although the testing apparatus used in different laboratories differs in detail, all investigators observe the same precautions.

The investigator must always be certain that ignition capability of sparks is being tested in the most easily ignited concentration of the gas or vapor used.

Once it has been established that the test apparatus yields the most easily ignited mixture, this fact need not be frequently reverified. However, when setting up new test apparatus, it is essential to verify by test that small changes in composition increase the required ignition energy. This is the only way to ensure that the means of introducing the mixture into the testing apparatus do not alter the composition of the test gas, and that the test gas is indeed of the most easily ignitable concentration.

The author, for example, for reasons of convenience, used

methanol vapor for testing the ignition capability of various sparks. Although the volume of the test chamber was known and an appropriate amount of methanol liquid to give the desired composition within the chamber after vaporization had been computed, the amount of liquid injected into the chamber was established empirically under the conditions of use. After initial adjustment of the feed apparatus there was little difficulty in maintaining the proper mixture, but this was occasionally checked by making slight perturbations in the amount of feed to determine that the ignition energy did in fact increase from a minimum value.

Where gases are being used it is, of course, much easier to control composition by filling reservoirs with appropriate partial pressures of the gas and air.

When gas– or vapor–air mixtures are stored in reservoirs and piped into the explosion chamber, it is especially important to eliminate leaks in the feed system by which the mixture can be diluted with air.

It is essential that all combustion products from a previous explosion or series of ignition attempts be completely removed by flushing the chamber with air or a clean gas mixture. If air is used, it too must be flushed from the chamber by an adequate flow of gas mixture.

Design and maintenance of a satisfactory contact mechanism is undoubtedly the most difficult problem facing anyone making ignition energy determinations. All experimenters have reported difficulty in obtaining reproducible results from electrode systems operated at voltage levels such that the electrodes are within the quenching distance. Although the author had some success several years ago with a rotating steel plate with a slot in it and a copper wire riding on the plate; and succeeded with relatively little difficulty in obtaining reproducible ignition data at levels comparable to that achieved by the break-spark apparatus used in United Kingdom, the wire needed frequent replacement. Most experimenters have found that high-melting-point wires are required to maintain stable geometry. Copper electrodes generally are unstable and need frequent replacement; the heat of arc formation causes the geometry of the copper electrode to change quickly. Platinum and tungsten electrodes are not as subject to this difficulty. There is no general rule except that unless apparatus is arranged so that for each ignition trial a new contact surface is presented, the calibration of the equipment must be frequently checked by determining the amount of energy which must be dissipated to ignite a known gas with known circuit conditions. Only in this way can one be assured that changing contact geometry or contamination of the contact surface has not altered the ignition capability of the test apparatus.

Even though gas composition is carefully controlled and the equipment successfully provides grossly stable electrode geometry, it is essential that changes in test conditions be related to changes in ignition energy only after numerous trials at each condition. British practice is to make 100 trials at the desired test condition.

In measuring the amount of energy required to ignite flammable mixtures in which contacts are closed to discharge capacitors, it is necessary that the contribution of energy from the power supply be nil. The need for concern in this regard would seem to be obvious. However, if data are being sought over several orders of magnitude of capacitance, and therefore over orders of magnitude of voltage, a resistor connected between the DC power supply and the test capacitor which satisfactorily isolates the low-voltage power supply when a large capacitor is short-circuited may be inappropriately small when small capacitors are charged to much higher voltages. The power supply may then cause current to flow in the arc, lowering the amount of stored energy required for ignition.

If the test apparatus operates on a fixed time cycle, too large an isolating resistor may so increase the time required to charge the capacitor to power-supply voltage that the capacitor is discharged at less than the desired voltage. Continuous monitoring of capacitor voltage could signal this problem, but it is best practice not to parallel the test capacitor with other circuit elements which might alter energy storage or release characteristics. If one is interested in relating energy stored in a capacitor to ignition, all the energy stored in the capacitor must be discharged into the arc. Any series inductance and resistance between the storage capacitor and the point of arcing will absorb energy, or lower the rate of energy discharge in the arc. The apparent stored energy required for ignition will be too high.

TYPICAL IGNITION TEST RESULTS

Figure 4-10a shows the results of typical tests of capacitive discharge ignition at low voltages. The shape of the energy-versus-

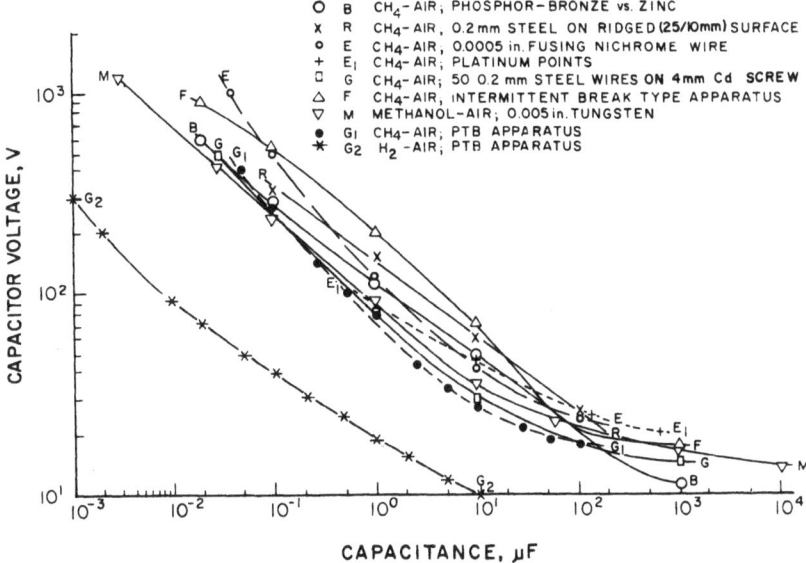

Fig. 4-10a. Low-voltage capacitor discharge ignition.

voltage curve is not at all unexpected, in view of the shape of the ignition curve which Lewis et al. found using pointed electrodes and relatively high-voltage discharge.   Because the electrodes are always within the quenching distance, as the voltage is lowered energy must be increased to compensate for increased quenching by the electrodes. Unfortunately, there is no analytical expression known to the author which adequately predicts the shape of the energy-versus-voltage curve.   The fact that for a given electrode geometry the required ignition energy increases as voltage is decreased is, however, in accord with our notions of quenching.

Some of the ignition characteristics plotted appear to be asymptotic to a voltage of 10–20 V. For a circuit entirely free of inductance this can be explained on the basis of the fact that the minimum short-arc voltage is of this magnitude and that circuit voltages below the minimum for the arc could not establish an arc to cause ignition. Only a small amount of lead inductance would be required, however, to raise the voltage above the minimum arc voltage, should there be a discontinuity in arc current, so that ignition at circuit voltages below the minimum arc voltage cannot be assumed to be

TABLE 4-2

Minimum Voltage (V) to Cause Ignition—8.3% CH$_4$

Capacitance		Circuit resistance, Ω					
		0	1	2	4	10	15
* 605		16	27	30	33	40	44
605		20	31	33	35	44	53
298	Electrolytic	21	33	34	36	46	55
170		23	34	35	37	48	56
116		25	34	37	38	48	57
49		28	35	39	39	48	56
* 100		16	28	31	36	44	50
97		21	32	36	38	46	56
50		23	32	37	39	48	58
19	Paper	29	36	40	41	51	60
10		42	51	54	55	63	74
* 2		60	72	76	84	94	104
* 1		88	106	126	146	–	–

*Pointed platinum electrodes. Others tested with point and a rod.

TABLE 4-3

Ignition Voltage (V), H$_2$–Air

Capacitance, μF	Resistance, Ω	
	0	100
1.0	25	220
8.0	17	160
66.0	12	170

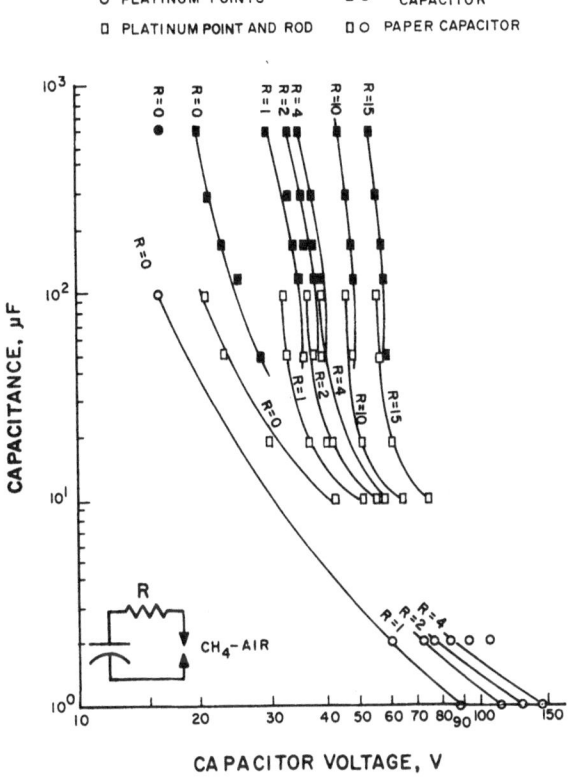

Fig. 4–10b. Effect of series resistance capacitor discharge ignition (from SMRE No. 107, p. 11).

impossible, even with closing contacts. In the author's opinion, it is also probable that ignition is caused by transfer of energy from the incipient arc in the vapor of the metal whisker or carbon particle volatilized at first contact, even though a steady state arc never forms.

EFFECT OF RESISTANCE IN DISCHARGE PATH

Table 4-2 gives the data obtained by Allsop and Guénault which show that moderate resistance in the capacitor's discharge path greatly increases the amount of energy which must be stored to cause ignition. Figure 4-10b is derived from these data.

TABLE 4-4

Ignition Voltage (V), H$_2$–Air

Capacitance,	Inductance, μH	
μF	2	85
1.0	150	250
8.0	45	75

The effects of series resistance and of series inductance for hydrogen–air ignition as reported by Müller are shown respectively in Tables 4-3 and 4-4. The method of ignition consisted of a pair of platinum wires, one stationary and one rotating, so fixed that closure occurred at 100 cm/sec.

EFFECTS OF ELECTRODE MATERIAL AND GEOMETRY

In connection with the experiments previously described, Allsop and Guénault determined the effects of changing electrode geometry and material. The data, as given in Table 4-5, do not lead to firm conclusions about the pertinent characteristcs of

TABLE 4-5

Changes in Ignition Voltage (V) with Changes in Shape and Material of Electrode

Electrode material and shape	Electrolytic capacitor			
	110 μF		605 μF	
	$R = 0$	$R = 1.0$	$R = 0$	$R = 1.0$
Platinum point to platinum rod	25	48	20	44
Platinum points	21	43	16	40
Steel point to steel rod	25	64	21	56
Steel points	23	53	20	46
Copper point to copper rod	26	61	21	56
Copper points	21	46	18	44
Blunt nichrome to carbon	46	70	–	–
Nichrome point to carbon (+)	29	66	23	58

electrode material, although they do substantiate previous statements about quenching. In all cases the voltage required for
ignition was less for two points than for a point and a rod.

OPENING CONTACTS IN INDUCTIVE AND RESISTIVE CIRCUITS

When a current-carrying circuit containing resistive or inductive
elements is broken, an arc may form at the contact point. If
sufficient energy is dissipated in the arc, ignition will occur. The
nature of the arc, the mechanism by which it forms and ignites
flammable material, is dependent upon the speed of break and the
circuit constants.

If electrodes in a very highly inductive circuit separate very
fast, the current attempts to fall instantaneously from its initial
value to zero. Since the contacts separate rapidly, the rate of
change of current, di/dt, is very high. The energy stored in the
inductor, L, is used to generate a voltage, $E = -L \, di/dt$, which attempts
to maintain the initial current flow. Even in circuits of fairly low
inductance it is possible to have transient voltages across opening
contacts in the order of kilovolts. In any case, when the inductance
is large enough and the speed of circuit break is high enough, the
back voltage produced by the inductance will be sufficient to break
down the gap. Breakdown of the gap may occur quite readily if
vaporization of contact material at the last contact point has
provided a source of ions which will conduct current. In many
cases, as the contacts first separate, a short arc with a typical
10-20 V drop is formed as a result of vaporization of the last
contact point. As the contacts separate further there is insufficient
voltage in the circuit to maintain the longer arc demanded by the
opening contacts; the arc dies, and current ceases to flow. This
in turn causes a high di/dt, and the stored energy in the inductor
causes a high voltage to appear across the gap, which breaks down.
This process may be repeated a few or many times, depending
upon the nature of the contacts, the speed of separation, and the
amount of energy stored in the inductor. The discharge in this
case may be short arc during its initial phases, may change to a
glow discharge with a drop of approximately 300 V, or may alternate
between the two.

In highly inductive circuits high breaking speeds are most

effective and will produce ignition with the least amount of stored energy. For many purposes it is sufficiently accurate, though somewhat conservative, to compute the energy stored in the inductor from the equation $W_1 = \frac{1}{2}LI^2$ and assume that all of the stored energy is dissipated in the arc or electrodes. Most often the ignition conditions are defined by specifying current and inductance. Since in fast-break and/or high-inductance circuits breakdown of the arc and release of the stored energy is determined by the rate of change of current, the value of the supply voltage in the circuit is relatively unimportant in determining the amount of energy required for ignition. Figure 4-14a shows that for inductances above approximately 0.1 H the curves for several voltage levels fall almost on top of one another. The voltage that can be generated across the contacts is frequently of order of kilovolts. Circuit voltage in instrument systems is usually small with respect to this value.

In circuits of low inductance and, in the limiting case, circuits with no inductance, formation of the arc is probably almost always caused by vaporization of the last point of contact causing the arc to form in metallic vapor. The arc will thereafter exist as long as there is sufficient circuit voltage to maintain the arc over the distance between the contacts as they open. The arc voltage will be no greater than the steady state short arc voltage, of the order of 10–20 V. This arc will last until the contacts are too far apart for the circuit voltage to maintain it.

In low-inductance circuits slow and intermittent contact operations are most efficient in producing ignition. Lower values of current are required with a slow or intermittent contact break than with a fast break. In circuits of low inductance, if the contacts open rapidly, the voltage produced by the change in current may not be great enough to break down the gap, and the arc which is produced by vaporization of the last contact point is rapidly extinguished as the contacts separate. If the contacts separate slowly, the arc persists for a longer time and there is greater opportunity to transfer energy to the surrounding flammable material.

Because this ignition mechanism is almost certainly a function of the life of the short arc the voltage in the circuit determines the contact separation when the arc is finally extinguished. This affects the amount of quenching by the contacts and length of time that energy is supplied to the flammable mixture and, therefore, determines the amount of current which must be broken to achieve ignition. Slow and intermittent break ignition in circuits of low inductance, therefore, show a very high degree of voltage dependence.

TEST EQUIPMENT FOR BREAK-SPARK IGNITION MEASUREMENT

By far the largest amount of data on ignition by break sparks has been published by investigators in Great Britain who have used the "Break-Spark" apparatus, which has been perfected in three stages during the past fifty years. The break-flash apparatus in its earliest form consisted of a pointed resilient strip of platinum which sprang against a platinum rod in such a fashion that the strip broke contact with the rod at high speed. In the original apparatus used by Wheeler, circa 1915, the platinum strip was stationary, while the rod revolved. In a later version, called Break-Flash Apparatus No. 1, the moving electrode was a strip of 10% iridium–platinum alloy tapering to a point, and at a still later date the strip was changed to platinum alloyed with molybdenum or ruthenium. The fixed electrode was a rod of platinum alloy 1.3 mm in diameter. In Break-Flash Apparatus No. 2 the electrodes between which the spark was produced were of the same shape and dimensions as in Apparatus No. 1. However, the strip electrode was bent into a smooth curve to make wiping contact with the rod, but with only the minimum pressure necessary to ensure a good electrical contact. Rapid break was produced by a spring mechanism and did not depend upon the elasticity of the strip. The whip of the strip still caused frequent fracture of the strip at its fixed end. It was also somewhat difficult to set the strip at exactly the proper curvature. The latest apparatus, Break-Flash No. 3, was designed to require less frequent adjustment of contacts and to provide easy control and measurement of the rate of electrode separation. Auxiliary circuits were also added to the machine to allow operation of other devices in synchronism with the break mechanism. Break-Flash Apparatus No. 3 is described in detail in Research Report No. 33 of the Safety in Mines Research Establishment. The rate of separation of the electrodes varies from 3–12 ft/sec. For official testing of intrinsically safe circuits, the device is adjusted to produce a rate of electrode separation of 7–8 ft/sec. When

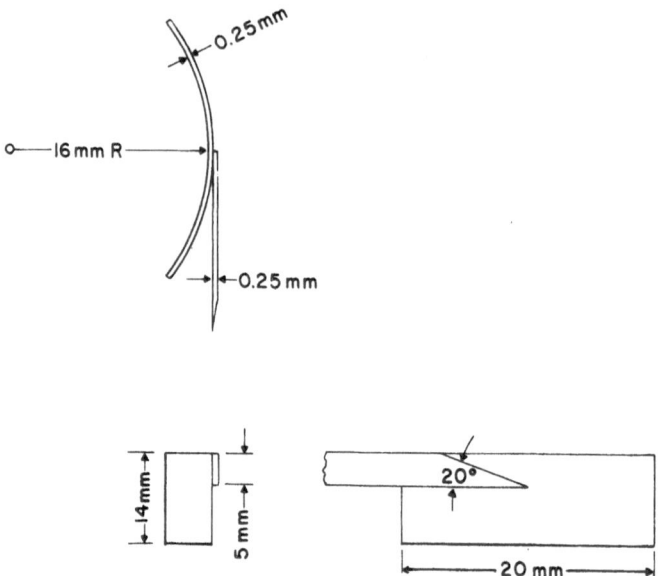

Fig. 4-11. Break-flash No. 3 electrodes.

breaking a circuit which includes a 0.095-H air core inductance, at least one ignition of an 8.3% methane–air mixture must be obtained in 100 trials at a current of 0.19 A, and no ignition must be obtained in 100 trials at a current of 0.18 A.

For circuits of low inductance the intermittent break apparatus may be used.

At PTB in Germany the rotating brush and counter-rotating slotted disc mechanism described earlier is also used for tests of inductive and resistive circuits.

The author, in some unpublished experiments, used a steel disc approximately 3 in. in diameter in which a 45° sector of the disc had been bent down. The fixed electrode, a copper wire, was allowed to rest on the disc, which rotated at 3600 rpm. The author found little difficulty in obtaining ignition of methanol vapors at energy levels consistent with those obtained by the British authorities in methane–air mixtures.

Several investigators have used various forms of breaking wire apparatus in which circuits are broken by placing wires under tension. The development of a British breaking wire apparatus is described in IEE Conference Report, Series No. 3 on "Flame-Proofing, Intrinsic Safety, and Other Safeguards in Electrical Instrument Practice." By placing wires of small diameter under tension it is possible to obtain ignition with break sparks at energy levels approaching those obtainable with high-voltage capacitive discharge methods. However, these results have no direct bearing on the problems of intrinsic safety in instrument systems, since break speeds as high as 1000 cm/sec produced by breaking wires under high initial tension are not at all representative of any situation likely to occur in a practical industrial system. Because the data obtained with such apparatus are not pertinent to the problems of intrinsic safety, and because the apparatus is suitable only for investigation of break-sparks, typical constructions will not be discussed further.

Figure 4-12 shows the relationship between circuit inductance and the current required to cause ignition by break-sparks, as reported by several laboratories.

The most thorough investigations of break-spark ignition and the effects of changing parameters has been carried out by the Safety in Mines Research Establishment, England. Many conclusions which can be drawn from their work on break-sparks are equally

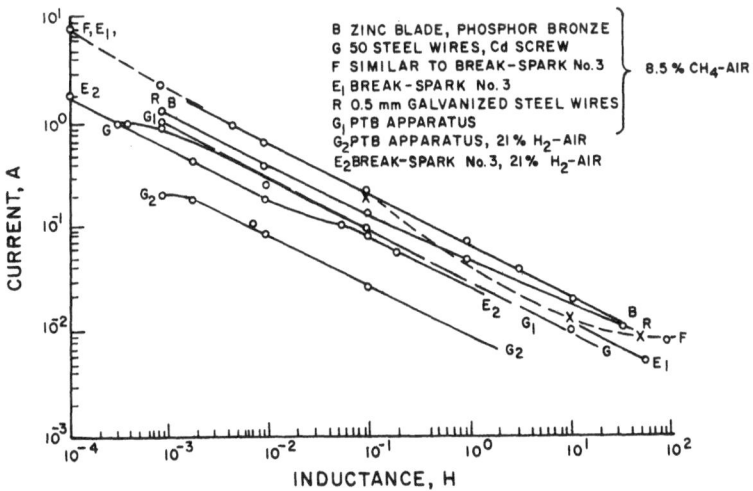

Fig. 4-12. Ignition data—inductive circuits.

pertinent to other modes of electrical ignition. The data are considered here because they were obtained with break-spark apparatus.

INFLUENCE OF CONTACT MATERIAL

In 1915 Thornton reported significant differences in ignition energy which he attributed to properties of the electrode material. His conclusions were in the main valid, but his arguments were sometimes forced and his supporting data crude by today's standards, so that they will not be reviewed in detail here. Wheeler, in 1926, again related the magnitude of igniting current to electrode material. Table 4-6 is derived from his data. The boiling points are taken from the 42nd Edition of the Handbook of Chemistry and Physics and differ greatly in some instances from those which he used.

Wheeler also recognized the relationship between characteristics of a short arc, electrode material, and ignition current required. He measured the duration of the arc and noted an apparent relation between boiling point of the metal and ease of maintaining the arc. Table 4-7 lists Wheeler's measured igniting currents and

TABLE 4-6

Igniting Current (A) vs. Electrode Material

8.35−8.55% Methane−Air, L = 31.75 mH

Metal	Boiling point, °C	Melting point, °C	Igniting current, A			
			First series			Second series
			80 V	100 V	120 V	120 V
Cadmium	767	321	—	—	0.22	0.23
Zinc	907	420	0.34	0.26	0.23	0.25
Silver	1950	961	0.44	0.41	0.38	0.32
Aluminum	2057	660	—	—	—	0.30
Tin	2270	232	0.66	0.53	0.45	—
Copper	2336	1083	—	—	0.49	0.38
Gold	2600	1063	0.86	0.59	0.50	0.34
Nickel	2900	1455	0.63	0.58	0.55	0.39
Iron	3000	1535	0.58	0.52	0.49	0.42
Platinum	4300	1774	0.65	0.56	0.48	0.48

TABLE 4-7

Igniting Current vs. Arc Characteristics

Material	Arc duration, sec	Igniting current, A	V_m , V	I_m , A
Cadmium	0.00321	0.23	11	0.1
Zinc	0.00234	0.25	10.5	0.1
Silver	—	0.32	12	0.4
Aluminum	—	0.30	14	—
Tin	—	0.36 (est.)	13.5	—
Copper	—	0.38	13	0.43
Gold	0.00070	0.34	15	0.38
Nickel	—	0.39	14	0.5
Iron	—	0.42	$13 - 15$	$0.35 - .55$
Platinum	0.00081	0.48	17.5	0.9

arc duration, and for comparison lists the minimum short-arc currents and voltages for these materials.

These comparisons point inescapably to the conclusion that electrode material plays an important role in determining ignition current, probably through dependence of arc characteristics on electrode material.

Further investigation by Guénault, however, although showing the effect of electrode material to be significant, also shows the relationship to be a more complex one than Wheeler or Thornton had supposed. As might be expected, in circuits of high inductance and fast break the influence of electrode material was nil. At lower inductances considerable differences in igniting current attributable to electrode material were noted. These differences were still more noticeable in slow-break tests. Figure 4-13 shows the influence of electrode material on igniting current in a slow break (0.5 in./sec), 24 V DC circuit. Guénault concluded that in circuits of high inductance the soft, easily oxidized, low-boiling-point materials required higher ignition current than platinum. In low-inductance circuits these materials allow ignition at lower current levels. He attributes the differences to the fact that in high-inductance circuits the discharge is a glow, while in high-current or low-inductance circuits the discharge is a short arc, much affected by electrode characteristics.

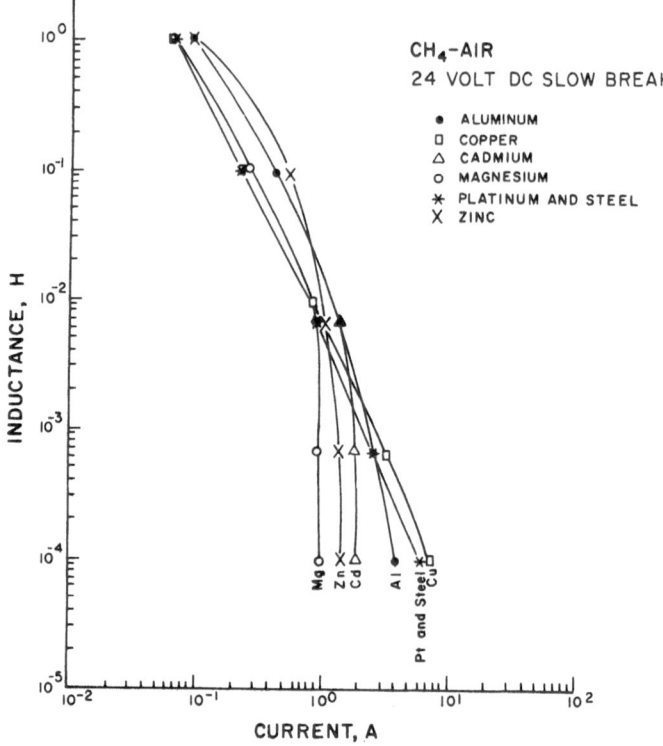

Fig. 4-13. Effect of electrode material (from SMRE No. 41).

INFLUENCE OF CIRCUIT VOLTAGE

It has already been noted that where circuit and mechanical conditions make $L\, di/dt$ large, the discharge voltage is high, and the contribution and characteristics of the electrodes are relatively unimportant. Similarly, if $L\, di/dt$ is large the circuit voltage is relatively unimportant in determining the magnitude of the ignition current.

Figure 4-14a shows the effect of circuit voltage on the current required to ignite 8.3% methane–air as determined by Guénault et al. for two different test equipments. One of them separated platinum–4% moly strip contacts at the rate of $32 \pm \frac{1}{2}$ in./sec; the other separated platinum–10% rhodium rods at 0.5 in./sec. These curves show the expected influence of circuit voltage. When inductance is high, circuit voltage has relatively little effect. In circuits of low inductance, voltage has a very pronounced effect on the amount of current required, the required current increasing rapidly as voltage is lowered. The effect of voltage variation is not remarkably different in the two sets of test apparatus.

Whether the circuit current is direct or alternating seems to make no difference in circuits of a few millihenries' inductance or greater. Figure 4-14b shows ignition currents measured using 24 V DC and 15 V AC in slow- and intermittent-break apparatus, as reported by Guénault et al.

In resistive circuits or "circuits of negligible inductance,"

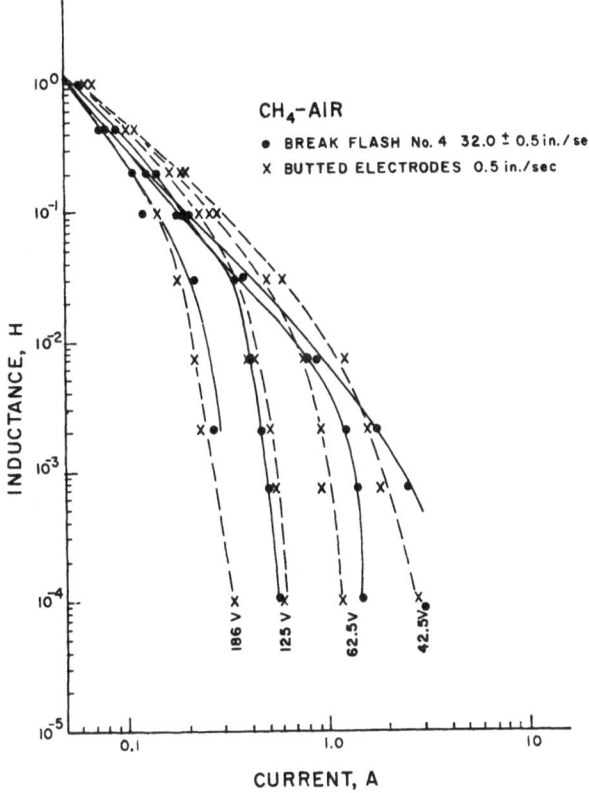

Fig. 4-14a. Effect of voltage on ignition current—slow and moderate speed (from SMRE No. 106, CH_4—Air).

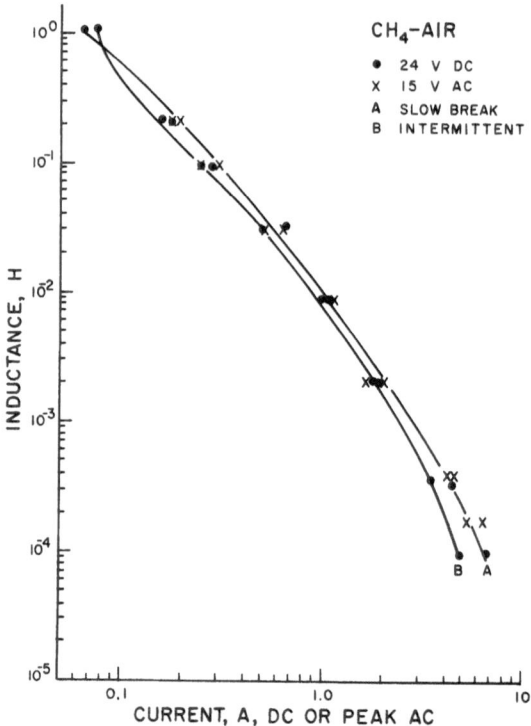

Fig. 4-14b. Comparison of AC and DC (from SMRE No. 106).

the relationship of greatest interest is that of the igniting current as a function of circuit voltage. Figure 4-14c shows data on resistive circuits derived from several sources. There is no easy way to rationalize differences between the curves from several sources. That the PTB apparatus ignites at lower currents is very likely caused by its use of cadmium for one electrode. The Belgian curve, based on a zinc blade against which a phosphor bronze contact is manually moved, is also low, probably because of the properties of the zinc electrode. The British data, derived from the investigation of Allsop, Guénault et al., using the intermittent break-spark apparatus, show odd and controversial cusps at 20 V and 200 V. The 20 V discontinuity, in the author's opinion, may represent a change in ignition mechanism from ignition by an arc discharge to ignition by a process analogous to hot-wire ignition. A platinum electrode system would have a

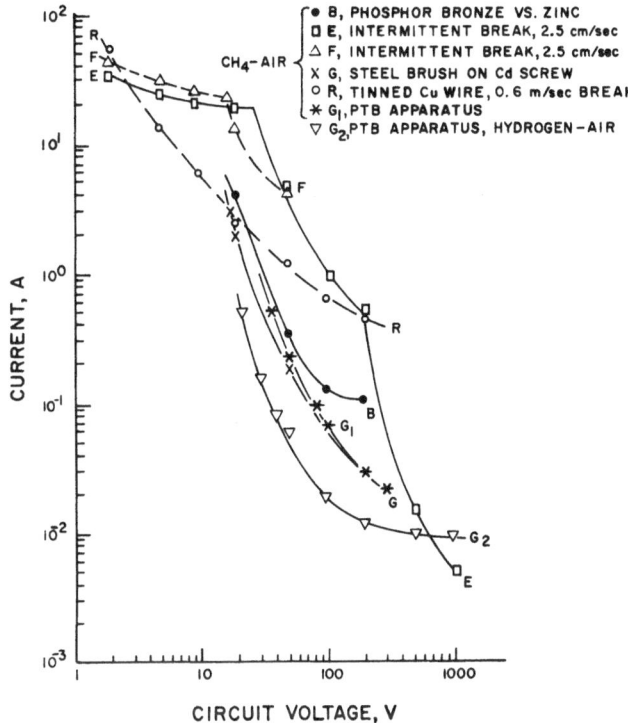

Fig. 4-14c. Ignition in resistive circuits.

minimum arc voltage of about 15 V. The same sharply rising ignition current is found in the German and Belgian data obtained with different test equipment. The discontinuity at 200 V can perhaps be attributed to transition from glow to arc discharge. Unfortunately, none of the other sources reported data above this level.

EFFECT OF SPEED OF CONTACT SEPARATION

In considering the effect of changing circuit voltage it was noted that whenever the mechanism of ignition and the circuit constants resulted in the inductive component of arc energy being large with respect to the contribution of the power supply in the circuit, the circuit voltage could change without changing the required igniting current. This section deals with essentially the same phenomenon,

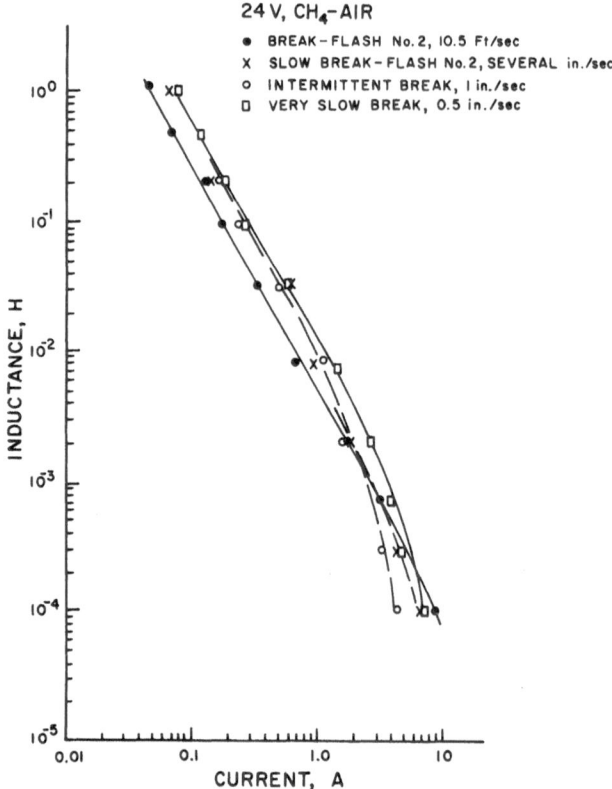

24 V, CH$_4$-AIR

● BREAK-FLASH No.2, 10.5 Ft/sec
X SLOW BREAK-FLASH No.2, SEVERAL in./sec
○ INTERMITTENT BREAK, 1 in./sec
□ VERY SLOW BREAK, 0.5 in./sec

Fig. 4-15. Effect of speed of break (from SMRE No. 106, 24 V, CH$_4$-Air).

except that the effect is considered of changing the speed while
holding the voltage constant. This effect is, of course, almost self-
evident from previous discussion. As the speed of break decreases,
the $L\ di/dt$ voltage decreases and, in circuits of moderate to high-
inductance, the required ignition current increases. At lower values
of inductance, where the ignition mechanism depends primarily on
energy transfer from a short arc, decreasing the speed of break
increases the time available to transfer energy to the flammable
material, and the required ignition current decreases.

Figure 4-15 illustrates the effect of changing the speed of
break in a circuit of 24V DC. The figure shows the relationship
between ignition current and inductance when the circuit is broken by
Break-Flash Apparatus No. 2, in which the contacts separated at

about 100 in./sec when spring operated, and at a few inches per second when operated manually. This comparison is of a single electrode system broken at different speeds. The other two curves show the relationship between inductance and ignition current for the Intermittent Break Apparatus previously described and an apparatus in which the electrodes separated at 0.5 in./sec. The contacts in this apparatus were butting 0.04-in. diameter platinum–10% rhodium alloy rods, operated by a cam. As expected, in the higher range of inductance the fast break is the most efficient mechanism, while for circuits of low inductance the slow or intermittent break is most hazardous.

IGNITION OF MATERIALS OTHER THAN METHANE

Because early interest in intrinsic safety in the United Kingdom stemmed from mine safety problems, most work was done with methane–air mixtures. Table I in British Standard 1259, March 1963, classified 126 materials, 49 of which had been ignition tested. The remainder were classified on the basis of similarity of chemical structure and properties to those which had been tested. The complete list of materials is included in Chapter 9. The basis for classificantion without testing lies in part in the following rationale, used by a committee of experts:

1. In a homologous series ignitability decreases as molecular weight increases, though the order may be reversed for one or two of the lower members of the series. In the case of the paraffin hydrocarbons propane is the most easily ignited.
2. Chlorination reduces ignitabilities.
3. Esters are slightly more difficult to ignite than the corresponding hydrocarbons.

Table 4-8a shows representative ignition data for materials which have been tested, as tabulated for the author by Mr. H. G. Riddlestone of the Electrical Research Association.

When minimum ignition energy is known it might seem reasonable that ignition current levels under less favorable conditions such as exist in the break-spark apparatus could be predicted. Table 4-8b shows break-spark ignition currents for a number of gases and vapors expressed as a ratio to the igniting current for

TABLE 4-8a

Minimum Igniting Currents (A) in 24-V Inductive Circuits

Compound	Inductance						Most ignitible concentration	
	0.102 mH	0.33 mH	0.825 mH	95 mH	~1.1 H	~15 H	%	mg/liter
Acetaldehyde	6.9		2.42	0.161	0.042	0.014		
Acetic acid			6.2	0.44	0.086			420
Acetone	6.5	3.9		0.165	0.045		9.0	
Acetylene	2.0		0.73	0.063	0.017	0.006	8.7	
Acrylonitrile			1.95	0.128	0.034			260
Allyl chloride			2.9	0.22	0.053			207
Allylene			1.5	0.113	0.032		6.7	
Ammonia				1.13	0.25		18.5	
Benzene	6.7			0.165	0.041	0.0135	5.5	178
Blue water gas		1.35		0.098	0.026	0.0073	31.0	
Butadiene	5.4		1.64	0.128	0.035	0.010	5.2	
Butane (calor gas)		3.7		0.170	0.043	0.0125	4.5	
Butene-2			2.6	0.149	0.042		5.5	
Butyl acetate			2.6	0.178	0.044			220
Butylamine			2.9	0.187	0.050			230
Carbon disulfide	1.52		0.75	0.064	0.022	0.008		730
Carbon monoxide	5.7	3.3		0.155	0.043	0.0135	51.0	
Chlorethane	7.6		3.0	0.195	0.051	0.017	7.25	
Chlorodimethyl-ether				0.161				537
Chloroethylene	6.9		2.4	0.166	0.049	0.015		
Cyclohexane	6.75			0.165	0.041	0.0135	8.5	128
Cyclohexene		3.4		0.160	0.042	0.0125		143
Cyclopropane	5.5		2.1	0.138	0.038	0.012	5.75	

Dibutyl ether			2.3	0.150	0.041			175
Diethyl ether	6.7		2.3	0.132	0.046			170
Dimethyl ether			2.0	0.140	0.036	0.012	8.0	
Epoxypropane			1.3	0.105	0.031			153
Ethyl mercaptan				0.148				210
Ethyl methyl ketone			2.5	0.151	0.041			200
Ethoxyethanol (cellosolve)			2.3	0.169	0.044			200
Ethylene	3.5			0.115	0.030	0.009	7.8	
Ethylene oxide	3.65		1.46	0.095	0.027	0.011	11.2	
Heptane	6.5	3.7		0.175	0.047			150
Hexane	6.1	3.6		0.165	0.043			122
Hydrogen	2.15	1.15		0.082	0.025	0.0067	22.0	
Isohexane	4.0	4.0		0.165	0.045	0.0135	3.4	400
Isopropyl nitrate	3.9		2.1	0.130	0.036			
Methane	7.0	3.9	2.5	0.165	0.043		8.3	
Methane*	6.4			0.157	0.044		8.9	
Methanol			2.4	0.162	0.046	0.013		215
Methyl acetate	8.3		2.59	0.178	0.043	0.015		315
Methyl acrylate				0.161		0.015		327
Nitromethane			2.6	0.151	0.045			540
Pentane	6.2			0.160	0.045			
Propane	6.1	3.8	2.2	0.148	0.039	0.012	3.9	
Propanol	6.7		2.4	0.151	0.048	0.014	5.25	210
Styrene		3.1		0.20	0.054			245
Town-gas	3.3			0.085	0.031	0.0075	14.0	
Trioxan		1.55	1.83	0.125	0.040			415

*Industrial: > 90% CH_4, < 10% H_2.

TABLE 4–8b

Comparison of Minimum Ignition Energy and Break-Spark Ignition Current

Flammable material	Minimum ignition energy W_m, mJ*	Ratio to methane, $W_m/W_{Methane}$	Calculated current ratio, $(W_m/W_{Methane})^{1/2}$	Measured ignition currents [Approximate inductance, H]								ERA source
				0.0001	0.002	0.02	0.095	0.2	0.5	1.0	14 †	
Hydrogen	0.019	0.068	0.26	0.26	0.23	0.28	0.44	0.42	0.49	0.49	0.45	D/T113
Ethylene	0.083	0.30	0.54	0.49	0.46	0.49	0.62	0.56	0.57	0.61	0.62	D/T106
Cyclo-propane	0.173	0.62	0.79	0.74	0.78	0.82	0.75	0.70	0.78	0.77	0.86	D/T126
Diethyl ether	0.198	0.71	0.84	0.91	0.72	0.74	0.71	0.85	—	0.94	0.83	D/T120
Hexane	0.24	0.86	0.93	0.86	0.83	—	0.89	0.78	—	0.87	—	G/T232
Heptane	0.24	0.86	0.93	0.91	0.77	—	0.95	—	—	0.94	—	G/T232
Propane	0.25	0.89	0.95	0.82	0.79	0.76	0.80	0.73	0.76	0.80	0.86	D/T126
Methane	0.28	1.00	1.00	1	1	1	1	1	1	1	1	D/T126

*Bureau of Mines Report 500 (High voltage, capacitive discharge).
†Iron Core.

methane under the same conditions. Although the ratio of measured currents tends to follow the pattern predicted from known minimum ignition energy values, there are some large deviations from the pattern, as in the values for hydrogen and propane for moderate (0.2–1.0 H) size inductances. In view of the fact that ignition energies or currents of several gases may not be in the same relationship for different methods of generating the igniting arc it is not surprising that when the mechanism of ignition is radically different, as in hot-wire ignition, the relative ease of ignition of the gases may appear to be quite different.

EFFECT OF SHUNT ELEMENTS ON IGNITION CURRENT

In an inductive circuit ignition by a break-spark is usually caused by an arc initiated and maintained from the stored energy of the inductance. After the circuit is broken the circuit appears as sketched below.

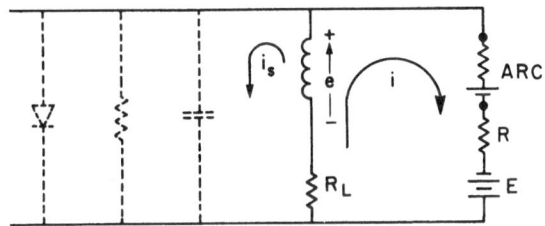

The voltage $e = -L\,di/dt$ is shown in a direction to strike and maintain the arc. The current at the moment before the circuit is broken would of course be $E/(R + R_L)$, where R includes all the resistance in the circuit except that of the inductor, R_L. After the circuit is broken the voltage e is driving current through the arc. The effect of connecting a resistor, a capacitor, or a nonlinear element such as a diode across the inductor can be seen qualitatively by considering the additional element to offer a path for current to flow in parallel with the arc. Not only does this steal energy from the arc, but a given voltage e at the inductor produces less voltage at the arc because the additional current in the shunt element increases the voltage drop in the inductor.

A numerical prediction of the effects of adding shunt elements will not be attempted here. The exact solution of the equations depends on adequately representing the V-I characteristics of the arc.

Qualitatively, though, consideration of the circuit sketched above can lead to the following conclusions:

1. If the shunt element draws current of significant size relative to the arc circuit the shunt element will significantly raise the initial current required for ignition.
2. If ignition without a shunt element was achieved by a high voltage breaking down the electrode gap to form one or more glow discharges with a 300-V drop in the arc, the addition of a shunt element would seem to be an effective way of reducing the voltage appearing at the inductor terminals.

The above conclusions are not independent. They represent two facets of the same situation. These conclusions, interpreted in terms of the ignition conditions before the shunt element was added, can be restated as follows:

1. The effectiveness of shunt elements in increasing the circuit current which must be broken to cause ignition will be greatest in high-speed and/or high-inductance circuits where the arc usually starts with a glow discharge, the currents broken are low, and the arc and circuit resistance R offer a relatively high impedance path compared to that of the shunt element.
2. In circuits of lower inductance or slow-break conditions, where igniting currents are high and ignition is caused by short, low-voltage arcs, shunt elements are less effective in raising the circuit current which must be broken because the impedance of the arc path is already quite low.

It has been observed that shunt capacitors, rather than increasing the initial circuit current, can cause the required ignition current to decrease if the circuit is broken slowly or intermittently. In the Safety in Mines Research Paper No. 106 shunt capacitance was shown to be quite effective in fast-break circuits. In slow- and intermittent-break circuits shunt capacitance decreased the required current to as low as 70% of the unshunted value.

Müller showed that shunting a 4-H inductor with capacitors increased the ignition current from 21 mA for $C = 0$ in a methane—

air mixture to 100 mA for $C = 0.25\mu$ F. Further increasing C to 10μ F decreased ignition current to 70 mA.

Unfortunately, the efficacy of shunt resistors and nonlinear elements in increasing the ignition current is, as was noted above, dependent on the fraction of the total circuit resistance contributed by the inductor resistance R_L. The data in Figures 4-16a-c can be used, therefore, only to indicate a representative degree of protection which can be attained by using shunt elements. Data on nonlinear elements are presented in a like manner. A larger selection and more convenient size of nonlinear elements are available for use today, but may or may not have equivalent effect in the circuit.

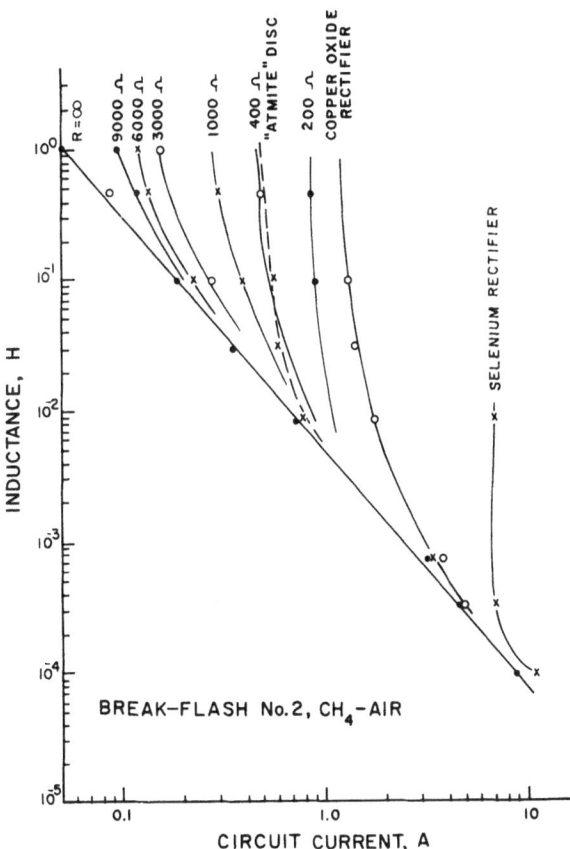

Fig. 4–16a. Effect of shunt elements (Break–Flash No. 2, CH_4–Air, from SMRE No. 106).

Figure 4-16a shows the effect of shunting resistors and non-linear elements in DC circuits broken by Break-Spark Apparatus No. 2.   Though resistors are effective in raising the ignition current, in a practical circuit where the current through the inductor is functional, there is a lower limit to the size of the shunt resistor.   A rectifier, however, does not shunt the inductor except with respect to voltages generated in it when the circuit is broken. In this case the rectifier resistance is low when protection is needed, high to current from the circuit source, and the degree of added safety is high compared to that obtainable using a resistive shunt of practical value.

Figure 4-16b illustrates the relative effectiveness of shunt

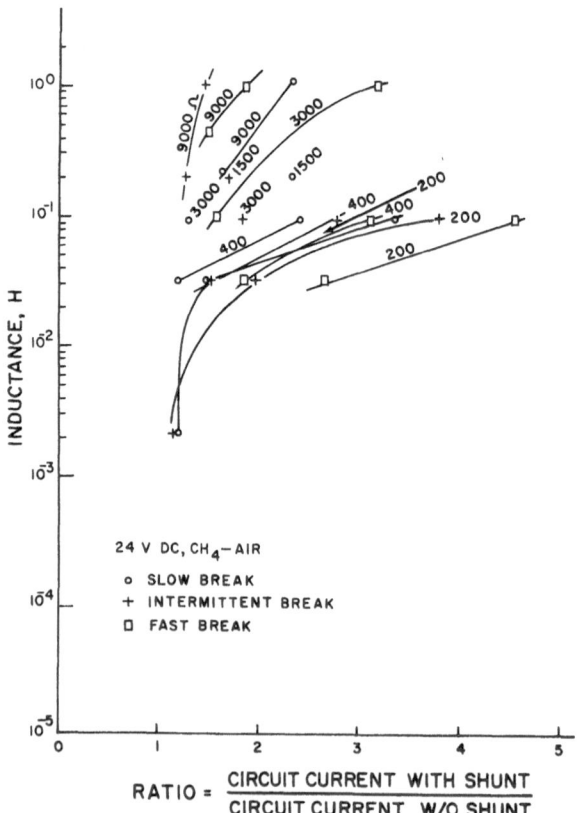

Fig. 4-16b. Influence of break speed on shunt effectiveness (from SMRE No. 106).

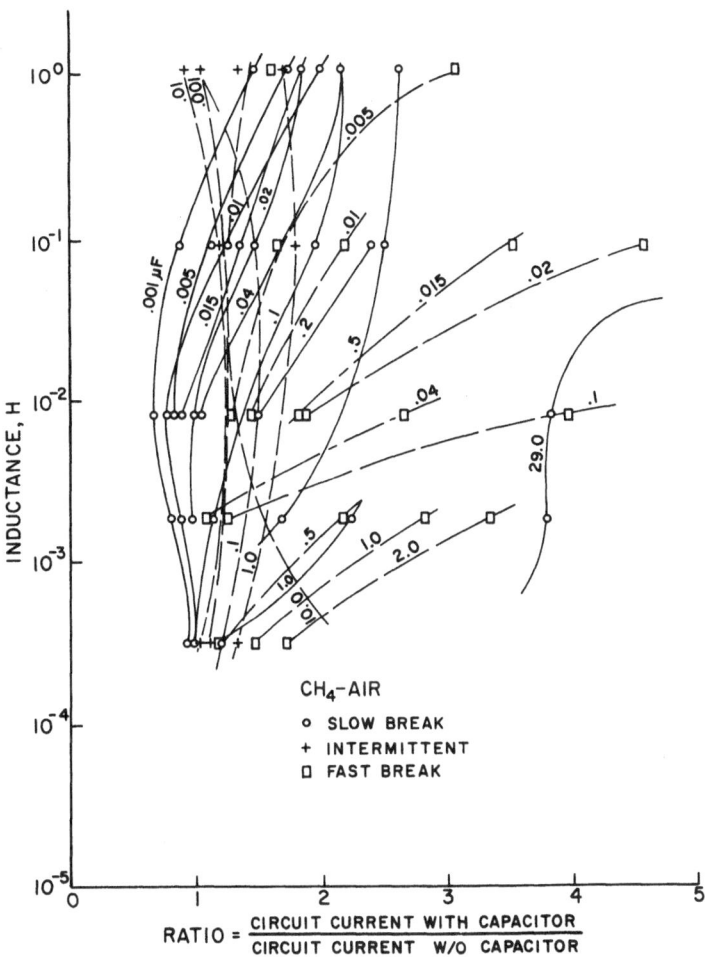

Fig. 4-16c. Effect of shunt capacitance—variation with break speed (from SMRE No. 106).

resistors in 24-V DC circuits with slow, intermittent, and fast break. Since the unshunted ignition currents decrease as the break mode is changed from "slow" to "intermittent" to " fast," the impedance of the circuit increases in that order. The effectiveness of a particular shunt resistance therefore increases as the rate of break is increased. This figure also shows, as does the preceding one, that the effectiveness of a given shunt decreases rapidly as the inductance of the circuit decreases.

Figure 4-16c shows, relative to unshunted ignition current, the effect of using capacitive shunts across inductors. Note that in some cases ignition current decreases.

HOT-WIRE IGNITION

It is universally recognized that a hot surface or a hot wire can ignite a flammable gas. Ignition by a sizable hot surface is the common method of determining ignition temperature of materials. However, there is little information available to define the limit conditions for hot-wire ignition.

The ignition mechanism of the hot wire differs from that of spark ignition in that the energy is imparted to the flammable mixture over an extended period of time, as compared with the 10^{-7}–10^{-6} sec during which energy is released from a high-voltage capacitor. In few cases is the time less than tens of milliseconds, making it relatively long compared to break-spark or low-voltage make-spark ignition. Because of the greater length of time during which energy is supplied, factors such as convection of the gas around the wire play an important part in making the mechanism relatively inefficient.

In the absence of convection currents one could postulate that a wire of diameter equal to the quenching diameter of the flammable mixture would ignite the mixture if its temperature were raised to the ignition temperature of the mixture. Such a wire would, in effect, start ignition above the critical diameter. Convection currents, however, may not allow a particular volume of gas to remain long enough in contact with the wire to reach ignition temperature unless the wire is at much higher temperature. When $4\frac{1}{2}$ in. long nickel bars, 0.040 in. thick and 0.5–1.0 in. wide, were heated to ignite 11% methane–air, the bar temperatures were 1079°C for the one-inch width and 1114°C for the 0.5-in. width. This is quite high relative to the ignition temperature of methane, 538°C.

If the wire diameter is decreased additional energy is required to bring the expanding wave front to the critical diameter D_q, and the required wire temperature is yet higher. The work of Stout and Jones indicated wire temperatures of 2000–2300°C. Thornton reported great difficulty in igniting methane with any wire whose melting point is below about 1800°C. Table 4-9 shows ignition currents for 30% hydrogen–air mixtures as reported by Thornton.

TABLE 4-9

Effect on Igniting Current, A, of Wire Diameter and Material

Material	Igniting current, A		
	Wire diameter 0.004 in.	Wire diameter 0.008 in.	Wire diameter 0.012 in.
Molybdenum	2.1 A	5.2 A	8.7 A
Tungsten	1.8	5.2	8.2
Silver	1.1	3.4	6.7
Gold	1.1	3.3	5.3
Nickel	1.4	3.3	5.2
Iron	1.1	2.8	4.5
Platinum	1.1	2.5	3.8

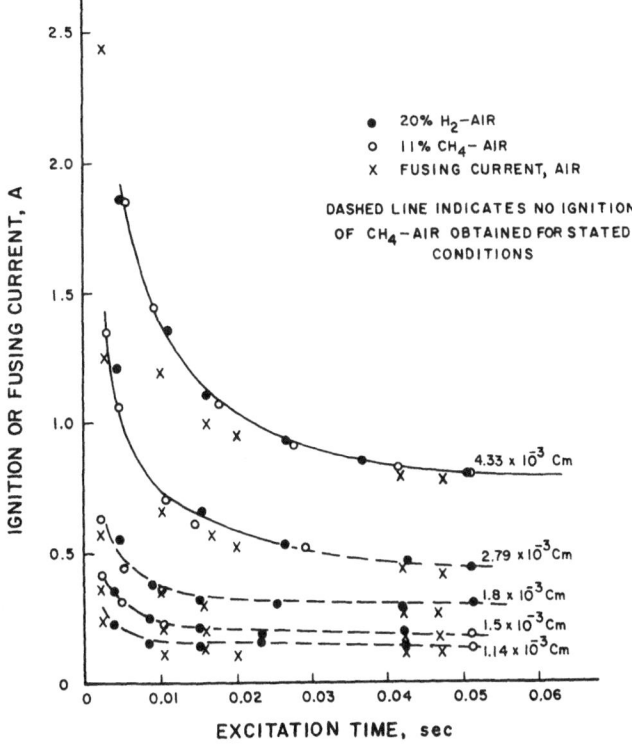

Fig. 4-17a. Hot-wire ignition (from Stout and Jones).

The wire sizes Thornton tested are all larger than 38-gauge, so that they are of a size, though of unlikely material, to be of practical interest to instrument people. It is interesting and significant to note that he found the smallest igniting current to be 1.1 A, which is less than the current required for break-spark ignition in many resistive circuits. It is therefore of real importance to decide whether hot-wire ignition is a mode of ignition which need be considered in evaluating and using instrument systems.

Stout and Jones presented data which show that some wires are so small that they cannot become sources of ignition. Although the Stout and Jones experiments were intended as a method of determining minimum ignition energy by extrapolating curves to zero time, the data can be used also for safety considerations by extrapolating to infinite time to determine the minimum current required

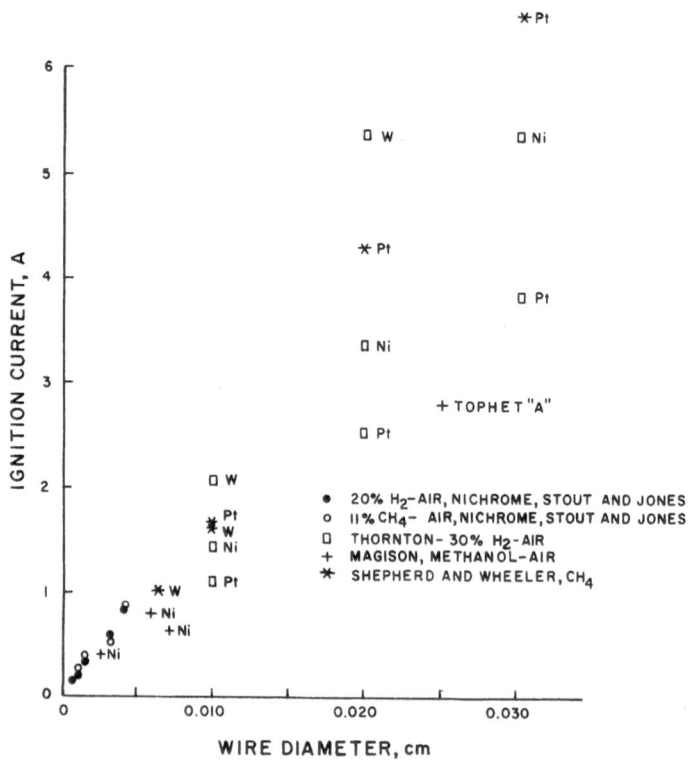

Fig. 4-17b. Ignition current vs. wire diameter.

for ignition. The data are plotted in Figure 4-17a. The $1.14 \cdot 10^{-3}$ cm diameter wire did not ignite the 11% methane–air mixture, though it ignited a 20% hydrogen–air mixture. Somewhat larger sizes caused ignition of methane–air only for relatively large currents applied for a short time. Smaller currents over a longer period of time are believed to have caused the wire to fuse before ignition. Figure 4-17b shows the current required to ignite various atmospheric mixtures as a function of wire size.

For a particular wire diameter, the current for hot-wire ignition is almost the same for methane–air and hydrogen–air mixtures and the igniting currents for both gases are not far removed from the currents required to fuse the wire. This suggests that ignition in many cases may be caused by the arc formed as the wire fused. This certainly would explain the sameness of ignition currents for mixtures of such widely different critical ignition energies. Most of the energy is required to melt the wire and form an arc. Only thereafter is the amount of energy related to gas properties.

The results of Stout and Jones, though interesting and applicable to any situation where high-melting-point wires may be used, still do not determine the fundamental importance of hot-wire ignition in the usual instrument construction. The author, in the work previously cited, reported a few measurements on copper and nickel wires which bear on this question. Using nickel wires of 0.001–0.010 in. diameter, we achieved ignition of methanol vapor at ignition currents comparable to those reported for methane and hydrogen by Thornton and Stout and Jones. These comparisons were made to verify an approximate equivalence in experimental technique. Straight copper wires 0.003 in. and 0.010 in. in diameter were found to fuse without causing an explosion. However, if the wire were looped it was possible to obtain an explosion with a current of 9 A if five loops were made in a 0.010-in. diameter wire. If only a half-loop were made in the wire, the wire would burn out without causing an explosion. The loops were approximately $\frac{1}{8}$ in. in diameter, of the sort which would be made in a heating element to concentrate thermal energy.

Other work, reported by Shepherd and Wheeler, was undertaken to determine the nature of the hazard from miners' lamps. These typically have 2-V, 0.65–1.0 A filaments. Shepherd and Wheeler found no difficulty in igniting methane–air mixtures by heating exposed filaments or by breaking the envelope of a lamp in a methane–air atmosphere. Ignition occurred even when the wire merely glowed dull red because oxidation of the tungsten filament raised its temperature.

In order to better understand the phenomenon, they heated platinum wires of 0.1, 0.2, and 0.3 mm diameter and tungsten wires of 0.065 mm and 0.1 mm diameter in a methane–air mixture. The igniting currents they obtained are plotted on Figure 4-17b. The plotted points represent suddenly applied currents. Other points plotted, except for those of Stout and Jones, represent gradually increased currents. Shepherd and Wheeler reasoned that failure to achieve ignition is enhanced by slow application of current which sets up strong convective air currents around the wire. Ignition may not result, but flameless combustion at the wire may raise wire temperature to the fusing point. Their report counsels rapid application of current in order to heat the surrounding gas before either strong convection currents are established or fusing occurs. They noted that as wire diameter is made smaller the ignition current approaches fusing current, indicating higher temperature for small sources, as reported by other workers. The 0.1-mm platinum wire fused in air at 1.95 A. In methane–air mixtures the fusing current decreased. In mixtures of concentration greater than 8.25%, 1.65 A, which ignited lower concentrations, fused the wire without ignition. These results are in apparent contradiction to those of Stout and Jones, but may be attributable to differences in wire material, platinum being somewhat catalytic. Shepherd and Wheeler attributed the decrease in fusing current to combustion on the surface of the wire. It is of more than passing interest that these authors report previous work by Wullner and Lehmann in 1886. These investigators had found that 0.15-mm wire would ignite mixtures less than 8.3% methane but fused without ignition in richer mixtures. With silver wires (no size reported) no ignition was obtained. With copper wire, ignition occurred occasionally when the wire fused.

Shepherd and Wheeler's data show that ignition by heated wires is not sharply dependent on concentration, as is spark-ignition. In general, rich mixtures of methane tended to cause small platinum wires to fuse without causing ignition. The 0.3-mm wire caused ignition at the same current over the range from 4.3% to 15.2% methane. The smaller wires caused ignition over a more restricted range of concentrations, but at the same current for all concentrations. A minimum igniting current at 8% methane concentration was observed with tungsten wire, but the igniting current increased only about 20% when concentration was changed to 5 or 12%.

Silver, in an excellent summary report, reviewed material from the sources already discussed, as well as from sources, including his own reports, which include the only extensive investigation of ignition by copper wires known to the author.

Silver reported an inability to ignite ether–air mixtures with fuse wires from 0.5, 1.0, and 5.0 A fuses at currents of 3.5–6 A in circuits of 4–8 V. Current was applied slowly. In other experiments Nos. 22, 28, and 34 copper wires heated for 1–90 sec at constant voltage did not ignite ether–air mixtures except when the Nos. 28 and 22 wires fused. Fusion alone was not a sufficient condition for ignition. Ignition occurred only when the wire fused less than 15 sec after voltage was applied. Ignition currents were 12.8 A for No. 28 wire and 45.8 A for No. 22 wire.

Ether–air and pentane–air mixtures were not ignited by Nos. 34, 36, or 37 copper wires heated slowly (1–15 min) from a constant current source. The exception was a No. 37 wire formed into a spiral and heated by 4 A.

Silver has also reported ignition of pentane–air mixtures by Nos. 28–42 copper wires heated from a constant-voltage source. These data also show that ignition is dependent on fusion of the copper conductor. For wires finer than No. 34, current at the instant of fusion was 4 A. For larger wires the current increased with wire diameter—to 12 A for No. 28 wire. Because these tests were made at constant voltage, initial current flow was significantly greater than the fusion current which produced ignition.

All the data on hot-wire ignition point to the following conclusions:

1. Ignition by fine wires will occur at current levels of a few amperes only if the wire material has a high melting point.
2. Ignition by copper wires is possible if currents are large enough to fuse the wire and greater than 4 A, or if the wire is coiled to concentrate heat.
3. In instruments hot-wire ignition need not be seriously considered unless fine wires of high-melting-point material can carry relatively high currents or unless wires of copper or

other low-melting-point material are coiled to concentrate heat. Except for these cases, ignition in circuits typical of instruments will occur because of break-sparks in resistive circuits at current levels less than those required for hot-wire ignition.

REFERENCES

1. Magison, E. C., "Low-Voltage Ignition of Hazardous Atmospheres," ISA Journal, July 1962.
2. Litchfield, E. L., "Minimum Ignition-Energy Concept and its Application to Safety Engineering," Bureau of Mines, RI 5671.
3. Vaillard, R., "Données relatives à l'inflamation des mélanges gazeux combustibles par l'étincelle électrique," Journal de Chimie Physique 40 (1943), pp. 101-108.
4. Morgan, J. D., "Principles of Ignition," Sir Isaac Pitman and Sons Ltd., London, 1942, p. 15.
5. Gehm, K. H., "Sonderschutzarten für den Explosionsschutz von elektrischen Betriebsmitteln," Elektro Welt, 1959, Nr. 10.
6. Muller, Kurt, "Eigensichere Stromkreise," Elektrotechnische Zeitschrift, 1 March 1957, p. 177-182.
7. Holm, R., "Electric Contacts Handbook," Springer-Verlag, Berlin, 1958.
8. Devins, J. C., and A. H. Sharbaugh, "The Fundamental Nature of Electrical Breakdown," Electro-Technology, Feb. 1961, pp. 103-122.
9. Lewis, B., and G. Von Elbe, "Combustion, Flames, and Explosions of Gases," 2nd Edition, pp. 323 ff., Academic Press.
10. Safety in Mines Research Paper No. 106, "Intrinsic Safety of Electrical Apparatus," 1947.
11. Safety in Mines Research Paper No. 107, "Exploders for Simultaneous Firing of Shots," 1950.
12. Safety in Mines Research Report No. 41, "Intrinsic Safety, A Resume of Recent Progress," 1952.
13. Safety in Mines Research Paper No. 104, "Intrinsic Safety of Electrical Apparatus," 1946.
14. Safety in Mines Research Report No. 33, "The Use of Break-Flash Apparatus No. 3 for Intrinsic Safety Testing," 1951.
15. Safety in Mines Research Board Paper No. 20, "The Electric Ignition of Firedamp," 1926.
16. McKinney, A. H., "Electrical Ignition of Combustible Atmospheres," Proceedings of 1960 Symposium on Safety for Electrical Instrumentation in Hazardous Areas, ISA, Pittsburgh.
17. Stout and Jones, "The Ignition of Gaseous Explosive Media by Hot Wires," 3rd Symposium on Combustion, Flame, and Explosion Phenomena, p. 329, Williams and Wilkins, 1949.
18. Shepherd, W. C. F., and R. V. Wheeler, "The Ignition of Gases by Hot Wires," Safety in Mines Research Board Paper No. 36, 1927.
19. IEE Conference Report Series No. 3, "Flame proofing, Intrinsic Safety, and Other Safeguards in Electrical Instrument Practice," 1962.
20. Silver, S., "A Review of the Ignition of Flammable Gases or Vapors by Hot Wires," Department of Mines and Technical Survey, Canada, Internal Report FMP-62/186-EEC, 1962.
21. Silver, S., "Tests of the Possibility of Ignition of Ether–Air Mixtures by the Melting of Small Fuse Wires," Department of Mines and Technical Surveys, Canada, Internal Report FMP-61/54-EEC, 1961.

22. Silver, S., and G. K. Brown, "Ignition of Pentane–Air Mixtures by Fusing Small-Diameter Copper Conductors in a Circuit of Low Inductance (22 μ H)," Department of Mines and Technical Survey, Canada, Fuels and Mining Practice Division Report FMP-64/157-EEC, 1964.

Chapter 5

Principles of Hazard Reduction

In this chapter the philosophy and the methods of reducing explosion hazard are summarized in very general terms. The aim is to establish a conceptual foundation for more detailed consideration of specific means of hazard reduction in the following chapters.

In most situations "reducing explosion hazard" means reducing the probability of significant damage as the result of an explosion. There are a variety of specific methods of accomplishing this. The diagram in Figure 5-1 shows the logical relationships among the methods. Not all the methods listed are common in instrument practice. Some are listed only for completeness.

The methods based on allowing ignition to occur depend upon ignition taking place under such well-controlled conditions that combustion does not cause significant damage. The use of an explosion-proof housing to contain an explosion and cool escaping gases so that combustion cannot spread beyond the enclosure is the most common technique of this sort in instrument practice. However, the use of a continuous source of ignition to localize combustion is quite commonplace in other contexts. If an ignition source is provided near the source of flammable material, ignition can be forced to take place within predetermined bounds where damage does not occur. The continuous pilot in gas appliances performs this function, confining combustion to the appliance by initiating combustion before a potentially hazardous uncontrolled volume of unburned gas has been liberated.

Those methods of reducing hazard which depend on preventing ignition are based on the fact that for an explosion to occur, two requirements must be met:

1. There must be combustible material present of proper con-

centration and adequate volume to support a self-propagating flame.

2. There must be available a source capable of imparting sufficient energy to the flammable material to cause ignition.

These two requirements must be met simultaneously. Failure to meet either requirement reduces the explosion hazard to zero.

METHODS BASED ON ELIMINATING THE SOURCE OF IGNITION

The most obvious way, and also in many cases the most sensible and most economical way, to eliminate the explosion hazard is to remove the source of ignition to an area where no hazard exists. This method is one of the first recognized in the National Electrical Code, Article 500.

The second method of eliminating hazard by eliminating the source of ignition is to apply the principle of intrinsic safety, also recognized in NEC, Article 500. Equipment and wiring which is intrinsically safe is incapable under normal or abnormal conditions of igniting a specified hazardous atmospheric mixture. Therefore, for practical purposes the source of ignition has been eliminated.

METHODS BASED ON CONTROLLING THE NATURE OF THE ATMOSPHERE AT THE IGNITION SOURCE

Preventing the Accumulation of Combustible Material in Explosive Concentration

The most common method of reducing hazard by preventing the combustible material from reaching explosive concentration is the use of purging or forced ventilation to prevent accumulation of a flammable atmosphere. However, it is also quite common to control concentration so that a mixture capable of supporting a self-propagating flame cannot exist. For example, in hydrogen annealing furnaces, the concentration of hydrogen is kept above the upper explosive limit. In hydrogen-cooled electrical generators the hydrogen concentration is also maintained well above the upper explosive limit. As long as the hydrogen concentration is above the upper explosive limit no self-sustained combustion can occur.

Another way of maintaining a noncombustible concentration is

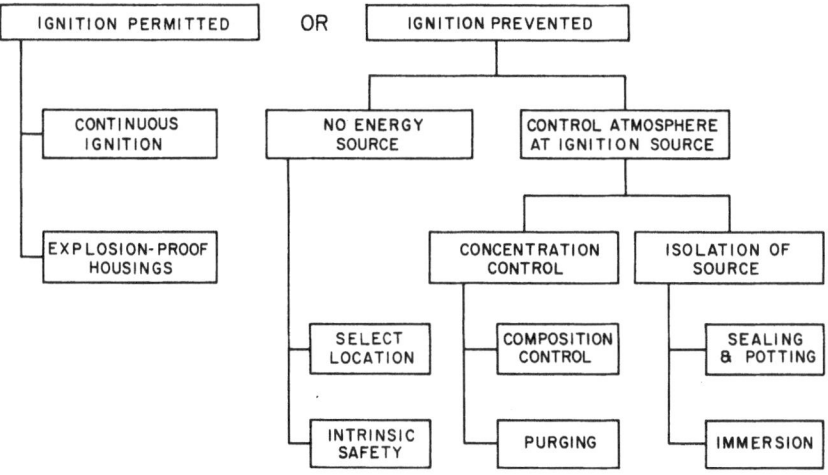

Fig. 5-1. Means of reducing explosion hazard.

to add inert material to the atmospheric mixture. In closed tanks, for example, carbon dioxide or nitrogen may be added to prevent the accumulation of combustible mixtures of vapor and air above the liquid surface. In coal mines, galleries and shafts may be rock-dusted to reduce the likelihood of coal dust explosions. In both cases the effect of adding inert material to the mixture is the same: the inert material adds thermal capacity without increasing the energy released by combustion and demands the addition of greater amounts of energy to raise the combustible elements of the atmosphere to their ignition temperature.

Isolating the Ignition Source From the Flammable Material

A technique which effectively prevents efficient contact between the ignition source and the flammable atmosphere is to immerse the ignition source in inert material such as oil or, as is done abroad, in sand. The function of the two materials is the same. Oil effectively prevents all contact between the combustible gas and the ignition source. Sand does not eliminate all contact because the sand is permeable to gases. However, the sand will so effectively quench any incipient flame that effective contact between atmosphere and source of ignition is impossible, and an explosion does not occur.

Hermetic or otherwise effective sealing, together with encapsulation, constitute two additional methods of eliminating effective contact between the source and the atmosphere.

THE DEGREE OF PROTECTION REQUIRED FOR DIFFERENT DEGREES OF HAZARD

The approach to hazard reduction taken in this book is a probabilistic approach—a statistical, though qualitative, approach such as is used in underwriting practice. It would be impossible to apply effectively any means of reducing hazard if one did not take this approach. The only alternative to a probabilistic approach is to consider all possible contingencies and eliminate all possible sources of hazard. For example, it is possible for you to be hit by an airplane as you read this sentence. It is certainly not probable, and for practical purposes you would certainly be willing to assume that you will not be killed by an airplace as you read.

The probability P_E that an explosion will occur is equal to the product of the probability P_c that combustible material is present and the probability P_I that sufficient ignition energy will be released. For example, if the ignition source is continuous, the probability P_I that the energy will be released is one; if a combustible material is present 1 hr in 10,000 hr the probability P_c is 0.0001 that the material is present in any one hour. The probability of an explosion, P_E, in any given hour is therefore $P_I \times P_c = 1 \times 0.0001 = 0.0001$. If the ignition source were present only one hour in every 10,000 hr the probability P_E of an explosion in any given hour would be $0.0001 \times 0.0001 = 10^{-8}$, or one in one hundred million. For almost any purpose a probability of 10^{-8} would be considered to be so low as to be essentially zero. Even a probability of 10^{-6} for a single event would be considered a good underwriting risk, one of essentially zero probability.

The presence of an atmosphere above the L. E. L. for one hour in 10,000 hr (one hour in thirteen months), as assumed above, is a more severe hazard than exists in most locations classified as Division 2. Presence of an ignition source for one hour in 10,000 is certainly a more severe hazard than is presented by recording potentiometers of conventional design. Even a probability P_E of 10^{-8} is therefore orders of magnitude greater than that which exists when a conventional instrument is installed a Division 2 location today.

On the other hand, if one expected that an atmosphere were to be above the L.E.L. as frequently as 1 hour in 1,000, strict rules to prevent entry of ignition sources would be enforced. Although the area would be classified Division 1, it would be far more hazardous than most Division 1 areas.

Area classification is not a quantitative procedure at the present time. The foregoing examples do not imply the existence of numerical criteria for classification of Division 1 and Division 2 locations. However, where the probability of the atmosphere being above the L. E. L. is as high as 0.001, most people would classify the location as Division 1 and act as though the area were nearly always hazardous, i.e., $P_c = 1$. In the paragraphs that follow a high probability is therefore represented by a probability of 1 for convenience of discussion. Similarly, a very low probability, less than 10^{-6}, is considered for convenience to be 0. Moderate or low probability therefore implies an absolute probability on the order of 10^{-4} to 10^{-6}.

The fundamental rule used in establishing the degree of protection which is required in a particular hazardous situation is that no single occurrence must raise the probability of explosion from zero to one, i.e., no one event shall significantly increase the hazard. This requirement is equivalent to stating that the probability of there being an explosion shall be essentially zero. The probability that two events each of low probability, say 10^{-4}, will occur simultaneously is 10^{-8} and may therefore for practical purposes be considered to be zero. Neither event alone raises the probability of an explosion to a high value.

If an atmosphere is above the L. E. L. frequently and the equipment in the atmosphere is not normally a source of ignition, the probability of explosion while the equipment is in normal working condition is effectively zero. If the equipment fails, releases a spark, and becomes a source of ignition—if the equipment fails even once per year—the probability of explosion in a given year would be undesirably high. A single occurrence of failure of the equipment raises the probability of explosion from a very low value to a very high one. A prudent individual would desire some additional protective means so that two failures of low probability—the failure of the equipment once per year and failure of the protective means—are required simultaneously in order that there be ignition of the flammable atmosphere. If this additional protective means is supplied, the probability of an explosion is effectively reduced to zero.

The foregoing is not a new philosophy. The rationale is implicit in the way in which the National Electrical Code defines area classifications. Although the definitions are not made in probabilistic terms, i.e., no probability numbers are specified, classification of a particular area as Division 1 or Division 2 is made primarily on the basis of loss experience, a consideration of the definitions in Article 500, and the judgment of the individual who is classifying the site:

1. A Division 1 area is one which is always, intermittently, or frequently hazardous, i.e., the probability is, in underwriting terms, "high" (though, as stated earlier, on an absolute basis the probability may be very low) that a flammable atmosphere will be present.

2. A Division 2 area is hazardous if the process equipment fails or if there is some other unexpected occurrence; according to underwriting criteria the probability that the atmosphere is hazardous in a Division 2 area is low. When process equipment is normally operating, it is nonhazardous, and becomes hazardous only if the equipment is in some abnormal condition.

3. An unclassified or nonhazardous area has zero probability that a flammable mixture will be present.

Equipment and wiring can be considered in a similar manner:

1. Intrinsically safe equipment is, by definition, equipment which is incapable of releasing sufficient energy under normal or abnormal conditions to ignite a specific hazardous atmospheric mixture. The probability of intrinsically safe equipment releasing sufficient energy to cause ignition is therefore zero.

2. Nonincendive equipment is equipment which, by definition, will not release sufficient energy in its normal working condition to ignite a specific hazardous atmospheric mixture. An ignition source is therefore not normally present. The probability is low that the equipment will fail and become ignition-capable.

3. Ignition-capable equipment is equipment which may have sparking contacts or hot surfaces which release sufficient energy in normal operation to ignite the flammable atmos-

Area Class Equipment Class	Division 1 $P_c = 1$	Division 2 $P_c -$ low	Nonhazardous $P_c = 0$
Intrinsically Safe $P_I \cong 0$	$P_E = 1 \times 0 = 0$ No Additional Safeguards	$P_E = 0$ (low) $= 0$ No Additional Safeguards	$P_E = 0 \times 0 = 0$ No Additional Safeguards
Nonincendive $P_I -$ low	$P_E = 1 \times$ (low) $=$ low One Additional Safeguard	$P_E =$ (low) $\times$ (low) $= 0$ No Additional Safeguards	$P_E = 0 \times$ (low) $= 0$ No Additional Safeguards
Ignition capable $P_I = 1$	$P_E = 1 \times 1 = 1$ Two Additional Safeguards	$P_E =$ (low) $\times 1 =$ low One Additional Safeguard	$P_E = 0 \times 1 = 0$ No Additional Safeguards

Fig. 5-2. Relationship between area and equipment classifications and required additional safeguards.

phere. Obviously, the probability of the ignition source being present in this case is one.

Figure 5-2 illustrates the possible combinations of the probability of the area being hazardous and the probability of the equipment being a source of ignition, in order to determine the probability of an explosion. The required number of additional safeguards to reduce the probability of an explosion effectively to zero is also shown.

As specific means of eliminating explosion hazard are considered in later chapters it will be seen that the installation and equipment recommendations are based on the principles presented above, i.e., no single event will raise the ignition probability from zero to one. The equivalent of two independent occurrences, each of low probability, is required.

However, one paradoxical situation exists. The National Electrical Code permits the use of ignition-capable equipment in a Division 1 area if it is enclosed in an explosion-proof housing. In accordance with the philosophy expounded in previous paragraphs, this would seem to be imprudent because a single failure, that of the explosion-proof housing, could cause the probability of explosion to rise from zero to one. One might therefore conclude that the use of explosion-proof housings in this manner is unsafe. In fact, however, this is not so; experience has proven it rather to be a safe practice. The apparent contradiction can be rationalized as follows. The fact that explosion-proof housings are designed with extremely conservative flame path and pressure test requirements constitutes in itself a safety factor considerably greater than that which may be considered minimum safe practice. Secondly, although in the foregoing discussion we have considered a Division 1 area to have unity probability of being hazardous, there are very few areas classified Division 1 which are hazardous even a small fraction of the time. If a significant portion of a processing plant were hazardous for extended periods of time, even if the electrical equipment were all de-energized, the probability of explosion from other causes, i.e., static electricity, sparks caused by tools, shoes, etc., is high. In support of this viewpoint is the fact that the L. E.L. of most gases and vapors is a much higher concentration than would be tolerable for prolonged exposure of human beings. Finally, most equipment installed in explosion-proof housings in Division 1 locations is not ignition-capable with a probability of 1 of igniting any atmosphere above the L. E.L. The product of all the probabilities therefore gives a probability of low absolute value.

REFERENCES

1. National Electrical Code, Articles 500 ff.
2. Maltby, F. L., "History of ISA Committee on Hazardous Area Instrumentation," Proceedings of 1960 Symposium on Safety for Electrical Instrumentation in Hazardous Areas, ISA, Pittsburgh.
3. Simons, Kögeler, Bijl, "Safety of Electrical Instruments in the Oil Industry," Institution of Electrical Engineers Paper No. 4001M, November 1962.
4. Hickes, W. F., "Intrinsic Safety," Proceedings of 1960 Symposium on Safety for Electrical Instrumentation in Hazardous Areas.
5. Recommended Practice RP12.1, "Electrical Instruments in Hazardous Atmospheres," Instrument Society of America, Pittsburgh.

Chapter 6

Explosion-Proof Housings

The use of explosion-proof housings is based on recognition of the fact that in many types of electrical equipment the amount of energy transferred to a combustible mixture during normal operation of the equipment or during probable and nonpreventable faults cannot in any way be reduced below that required for ignition. One way in which such equipment can be used safely in a hazardous location is to provide an enclosure so constructed that, if ignition does occur around the equipment, the flame cannot propagate outside the enclosure and spread to the surrounding atmosphere. For the enclosure to perform this function it must c o n t a i n the internal explosion without damage and c o o l any gases which escape so that they cannot ignite a flammable mixture surrounding the enclosure.

Explosion-proof enclosures are not vapor-tight. It is expected that gas or vapor will enter the enclosure and be ignited if there is an ignition source. The pressure developed inside an industrial explosion-proof enclosure is less than the pressure measured in a completely sealed container in the laboratory. In closed vessels, where leakage from the vessel is prevented, explosion pressures of typical Group C and D materials range to 130 psi, with some as high as 155 psi. In a practical explosion-proof housing the pressures are somewhat less because expanding gases escape through the joints.

The effectiveness of joint leakage in reducing the explosion pressure from that attained in a sealed chamber is less with fast-burning gases like hydrogen than with slow-burning gases like methane. Figure 6-1 is drawn from Ministry of Fuel and Power data. The bold lines show the maximum permissible gap for 1-in. flanges according to British Standard 229. No permissible gap has been established for hydrogen.

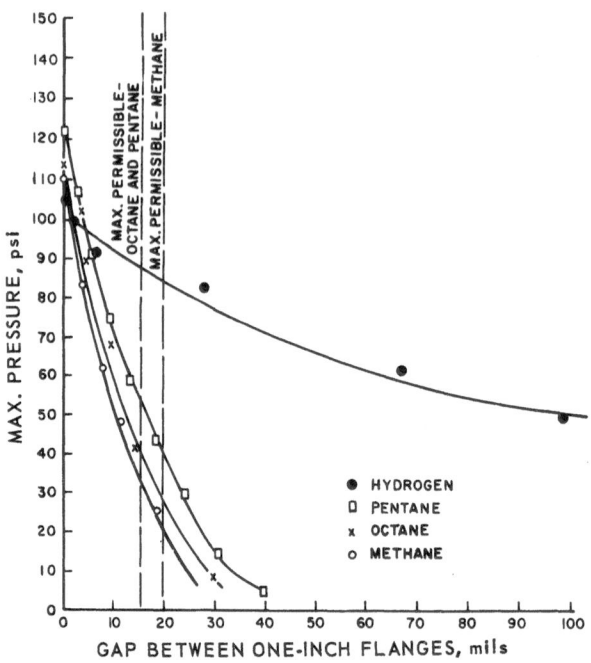

Fig. 6-1. Reduction of maximum explosion pressure by gaps (from SMRE Review, 1944).

It must be noted that under some conditions it is quite possible to develop explosion pressures considerably higher than those found in even completely closed vessels. Pressures on the order of 500 psi have been measured in rotating machinery. However, the volumes and the conditions of test are not at all comparable to those usually of interest to instrument manufacturers and users. In rotating machinery the considerably higher pressures may be caused by pressure piling and by detonation. Pressure piling occurs when the expanding combustion wave precompresses the unburned gases. In rotating machinery, for example, the volume of one end bell is connected to the volume of the other end bell by means of relatively small clearance between the rotor and stator or by connecting passages through the rotor or stator structure. In electrical installations there may be a similar situation between two cases connected by conduit. If an explosion occurs in one of the cases, the combustion wave attempts to expand into the conduit and the second case. The gas in the connecting conduit and other case is precompressed by thermal expansion of the gases in the first case before flame arives to cause ignition. The explosion pressure after ignition occurs is therefore considerably higher than the normal explosion pressure because of the precompression. Not only are the absolute explosion pressures higher, but the rate of change of pressure is higher. As unburned gas ahead of the advancing combustion wave is compressed, its temperature is raised. Much less energy must be extracted from the approaching combustion wave to raise a new layer of this preheated gas to the ignition temperature and the flame, therefore, propagates at a faster rate.

If as a flame propagates, interaction between the combustion wave and conduit walls produces turbulence and enhanced mixing, further increased flame speed may produce shock waves which will propagate through the conduit, reflecting off the walls and further increasing turbulence at points of interaction between the shock wave and combustion wave. This results in transition from a thermal combustion wave to a detonation wave. Velocity increases from tens of feet per second to hundreds or even thousands of feet per second. The prime requisite for transition from a combustion wave to a detonation wave in situations of interest to instrument users is the existence of a tube or conduit of length many times the diameter. Conduit connecting explosion-proof housings fits this requirement remarkably well, and it is partially out of concern for pressure piling and detonation that the National Electrical Code stipulates that conduit entering or leaving most explosion-proof housings be suitably sealed. In rotating machinery mixing and compression of gases is aided by mechanical rotation, and higher flame speeds and detonation may occur.

In Chapter 3 the effect of cool surfaces on the development of a combustion flame was considered. One might expect that if an explosion-proof chamber were constructed with flanged joints and the gap width in the joint were equal to the quenching distance, this flanged joint would cool the flame and prevent the combustion wave from propagating outside the enclosure. From a qualitative standpoint this rationale is correct. Quantitatively, however, it is too optimistic because of the hot, expanding combustion products inside the enclosure. Pressure inside the enclosure is higher than the pressure outside the enclosure. The speed of the jet issuing from the enclosure may therefore be higher than the speed of a freely developing combustion wave and a gap of quenching dimension will not cool the escaping gas sufficiently. More importantly, it is not necessary that a combustion wave (flame) be propagated through the gap in order to ignite the atmosphere surrounding the enclosure. It is only necessary that burned gases at a temperature somewhat higher than the ignition temperature of the mixture outside be communicated. Because the ignition temperatures of most gases or vapors in air are in the range 100–600°C, but flame temperatures are 1500–2000°C, the allowable gap width is considerably less than the quenching distance measured in electrical ignition experiments.

The manner in which ignition by the escaping jet occurs is presumed at the present time to be as follows. When an explosion occurs inside the explosion-proof chamber the combustion wave propagates outward to the walls of the chamber, burning all of the available combustible material inside the chamber and raising both pressure and temperature. The burned gas, heated and under pressure, is now forced out through the gap between the flanges of the explosion-proof housing. This jet of burned gas starts out through the flange at a temperature on the order of 1500–2000°C, is cooled by the flange, and then issues into the surrounding combustible atmosphere. As the jet enters the surrounding atmosphere, combustible material is entrained in the jet. The entry and mixing of this combustible material into the jet provides fuel for combustion outside the chamber. It also cools the jet below the temperature at which it issued from the gap. If the rate of issuance of material and the temperature are sufficiently high, combustible material will enter the jet without cooling the jet below the ignition temperature of the flammable gas, and the atmosphere external to the explosion-proof housing will be ignited. From this one could conclude that if the flanges of an explosion-proof housing were preheated to temperatures near the ignition temperature of the gas external to the housing, the safe distance between these flanges would approach zero. This hypothesis has been validated by test. One could also assume that if high amounts of water vapor were contained in the gas surrounding the explosion-proof housing, this would increase the amount of cooling of the jet and, other conditions being equal, would increase the allowable safe gap width. This assumption is also valid. The relationship between gap width and the nature of the flammable materials inside and outside the enclosure can also be qualitatively estimated from this approach. Hydrogen has a very high flame temperature; therefore, the temperature of the burned gases escaping through a given gap will be relatively high.

A hydrogen—air mixture external to the housing requires relatively low additional energy to cause ignition. These two factors in combination could lead one to expect a considerably narrower safe gap for hydrogen—air flames than for a gas such as methane which has a much lower flame temperature and higher ignition energy. Such is indeed the case. The safe gap for methane between one-inch-wide flanges is defined for practical use as 0.020 in. in British Standard 229. The safe gap for hydrogen was found to be so small as to be impractical to maintain. (This is not a universal view. Housings suitable for hydrogen are approved in the U. S. and Germany. Maintenance of 0.0015-in. gaps between flanges is common in the U. S.)

Porous plugs or screens are occasionally used to vent a housing and minimize pressure rise inside the enclosure. The theory of operation of porous plugs and screens is similar to that for the safe gap width. However, as more of the explosion-proof housing wall is replaced by porous plugs and vents, the maximum pressure attained in the housing when explosion occurs decreases. As the pressure approaches atmospheric the propagation of the flame (combustion wave) more nearly approaches the propagation of the wave in an unbounded large chamber. The diameter of holes in protective screens, as in the famous Davy lamp, approaches that which would be predicted from quenching distances determined in ignition experiments. The quenching distance for methane of most easily ignited concentrations is 0.080 in. Davy recommended gauze made of 0.016 in—0.025 in. diameter iron wire spaced 28 wires to the inch, but found 0.014-in. diameter wire spaced 25 to the inch also to be safe. Though the apertures in these gauzes are still small compared to the quenching distance, they are of the same size as gaps permitted with 1-in. wide flanges in United Kingdom.

The establishment of maximum safe gaps or the testing of a proposed explosion-proof housing for safety is still very much an empirical matter. In the United Kingdom the chamber to be tested is filled with the most incendive mixture of the test gas, i.e., the gas mixture which will ignite the most easily ignited concentration outside the chamber through the smallest gap; and the atmosphere surrounding the chamber is the most easily ignited mixture of the gas. When the combustible mixture inside the chamber is ignited, the housing must withstand the effects of the explosion without deformation or damage and the mixture outside the chamber must not ignite. There must of course be no sign of flame. At Underwriters' Laboratories a series of tests is performed over a range of concentrations bracketing the mixture which produces the highest explosion pressure. The mixture inside and outside the enclosure is the same.

DESIGN CRITERIA, UNITED STATES AND CANADA

The following design criteria for Class 1, Group D equipment are summarized from Underwriters' Laboratories Standard No. 698 and CSA Standard C130. This material is presented for didactic purposes. It is not intended as a substitute for study of the latest issues of the source documents to determine specific requirements. The requirements summarized below are, of course, supplementary to the requirements for ordinary locations.

1. Materials

Enclosures, except for windows, must be of substantial metallic construction, must completely encase the electrical assembly and all electrical connections, and must be designed to withstand the normal conditions of use in the industry and for the purpose intended.

Windows may be of glass or other material acceptable to the purpose which, "in its mounting, can withstand the impact of a 4-lb weight falling 6 in. the point of impact being a hardened steel ball, 1 in. in diameter." (Portion in quotes is from C130.)

2. Strength

UL 698. The enclosure must be able to withstand without rupture or permanent deformation a hydrostatic test of four times the maximum pressure which is developed within the enclosure during an actual explosion test. Enclosed chamber pressures of 75 to 150 psi are typical, although the actual pressure is affected by size, shape, the combustible mixture used, and the arrangement of equipment within the case. An exception to the hydrostatic test may be made if acceptable calculations show a factor of safety of five based on the maximum pressure developed during the explosion test. If the material of construction is rolled steel, then no permanent deformation should be observed during a hydrostatic test at a pressure two times the maximum observed during the explosion test, and there should be no rupture at three times the maximum observed test pressure.

CSA Standard C130. Instead of basing the hydrostatic test pressure on the maximum observed explosion test pressure, Canadian authorities define a reference pressure, the defined internal explosion pressure (DIEP), and give it a value of 140 psi based on a background of Class I, Group C and D explosion tests.

Hydrostatic tests are to be conducted at a pressure of four times DIEP if the enclosure is cast metal and three times DIEP if the enclosure is fabricated rolled metal.

3. Joints

Joints shall be metal-to-metal, flat, stepped, or threaded. Joint width shall be not less than $\frac{3}{4}$ in. except that an enclosure having an internal volume of 300 in.^{3} or less may have $\frac{3}{8}$-in. wide flanges in Canada or $\frac{1}{2}$-in. rabbet joints in the U. S. Enclosures with $\frac{3}{8}$-in. thick flanges and internal volume of 300 in.^{3} or less will be accepted for test by U.L. Underwriters' Laboratories will also accept for test $\frac{1}{4}$-in. wide flanges with 0.005-in. gaps if explosion-proof vents limit the explosion pressure rise to 5 psi.

When joints are bolted the following criteria must be met: $\frac{3}{8}$-in. wide joints must not accept a 0.0015 feeler more than $\frac{1}{8}$ in.; $\frac{3}{4}$-in. wide joints must have a gap of 0.002 in. or less. Wider joints may have gaps increasing at 0.00125 in. per $\frac{1}{4}$ in. increased width to a maximum gap of 0.0045 in. at 1.25 in. joint width.

4. Bolt Spacing and Location

The Canadian Standard requires that if the bolt hole is within the required joint width, the distance from the inside of the enclosure to the bolt hole edge shall be $\frac{3}{8}$ in. minimum, and the bolt hole diameter shall be not more than $\frac{1}{32}$ in. greater than the bolt diameter.

Underwriters' Laboratories stipulates the minimum distance to the bolt hole edge to be $\frac{1}{2}$ in., and also requires the flange thickness to the bottom of the bolt head to be at least one-half the joint width. If the bolt hole is to be counted as part of the flame path, it shall not be more than $\frac{1}{32}$ in. larger in diameter than the bolt.

5. Shaft Clearances

Machined shafts for making adjustments, etc., shall have path length of at least 1 in. Diametral clearance shall be not larger than 0.003 in. (U.L. says 0.0033 in.) and may be increased to 0.004 in. for $1\frac{1}{8}$ in. path length or 0.0045 in. for $1\frac{1}{4}$ in. path length.

Threaded joints shall have 5 full thread engagement. CSA specifies Class I fit.

6. Holes

Holes in the enclosure for securing the nameplate or a mechanism must be bottomed or closed by welding or must have not less than five threads, with the entering threaded part secured against removal by staking, welding, riveting, or other substantial means of locking.

Removable bolts or screws may not extend through the enclosure wall. Metal thickness at the bottom of the hole shall be the larger of $\frac{1}{8}$ in. or one-third the hole diameter.

7. Connections

All connections shall be designed to permit 5 full thread engagement of rigid conduit. Unused openings must be sealed with pipe plugs having not less than five-thread engagement.

8. Temperature Rise

Exterior observable temperatures, based on 40°C ambient, shall not exceed: (Group C) 180°C, or 356°F; (Group D) 280°C, or 536°F.

9. Marking

In addition to other markings which may be required, a warning nameplate must be affixed carrying the following statement or an approved substitute: "This apparatus must be disconnected from the supplying circuit before opening and must be tightly closed again before it is put into operation. See instruction book."

TESTING

In the testing of explosion-proof enclosures and their listing by Underwriters' Laboratories, it is presumed that the equipment to be used within the enclosure is installed in its normal manner during the test.   In doing so, U.L. recognizes that equipment could be installed within an enclosure in a way to greatly modify the distribution of the free volume and cause pressure piling, which would vitiate any listing granted on the enclosure tested either empty or with other equipment. However, a sizable proportion of the enclosures currently being sold are not listed by Underwriters' Laboratories.   Many are designed and constructed on the basis of UL Document 698 and hydrostatically tested in accordance with those requirements.   Others are designed on the basis of previous experience with hydrostatic or explosion tests.   In either case the safety of these enclosures is certainly more than adequate. Hydrostatic testing imposes a factor-of-4 safety in pressure in addition to any reduction in hazard by venting. The gaps specified in UL 698 are quite conservative, as will be seen when considering British practice.

DESIGN CRITERIA IN THE UNITED KINGDOM

The material presented below is summarized from British Standard 229 for the flame-proof enclosure of electrical apparatus. This information is presented because, although mechanical design of British flameproof enclosures is not necessarily acceptable to authorities in all European countries, the gap requirements are indicative of those of European requirements, and of the requirements of IEC 79, the International Standard on Flameproof Enclosures. The specific requirements, however, differ from country to country, and IEC 79 is being revised.

The requirements for British flameproof enclosures and the classification of gases and vapors are based on tests started in 1922 to determine minimum safe gaps. The safe gap was determined by using a bronze sphere with explosive mixture inside and out, arranged so that the gap size could be altered until the gap width was found which would not allow ignition of the external atmosphere. For a particular gap the test procedure was to measure the percentage of ignition trials in which there was ignition of the external gas. These data on percent ignition related to gap width were used to derive a statistical safe gap from the experimental safe gap data. From the statistical safe gap, using a multiplier of approximately 0.6, the permissible safe gap was derived. There is one chance in one thousand that the statistical safe gap is greater than the gap for which the risk of ignition is one in 10^6. The factor of 0.6 is used to account for possibility of incorrect aligment of the flanges, mechanical damage, and other unpredictable factors.

Classification of Gases and Vapors Based on Statistical Safe Gap

The classification of gases and vapors for consideration of flameproof enclosures in the United Kingdom results in a grouping not unlike the classification into groups A, B, C, and D in the National Electrical Code. The classification used in the United Kingdom is given in Table 6-1.

Permissible Safe Gaps

Based on the above statistical safe gaps and further classification of the equipment, permissible safe gaps have been established, as summarized in Table 6-2.

The subclasses used in Table 6-2 are defined as follows:

A(i). . . joints and shaft clearances for 1-in. length in housings which would normally be air-filled.

A(ii) . . diametral clearance for the shafts of motors and generators which do not have labyrinth seals.

A(iii). . joint clearance for $\frac{1}{2}$-in. flanges in housings which are normally air-filled.

TABLE 6-1

Classification of Gases and Vapors for Consideration of Flameproof Enclosures

Group	Typical vapors and gases	Statistical safe gap (in.)	
		1-in. flange	$\frac{1}{2}$-in. flange
I	methane	0.0340	0.020
II	propane, butane, and other hydrocarbons	0.0250	0.014
III a	ethylene, diethyl ether, ethylene oxide	0.015 −0.025	0.012 −0.014
III b	coal gas and coke oven gas	0.015 −0.025	none
IV	acetylene, carbon disulfide, water gas, hydrogen, ethyl nitrate	0 −0.015	none

TABLE 6-2

British Classification of Permissible Safe Gaps (in.)

Group	1-in. flange			½-in. flange
	Class A (i)	Class A (ii)	Class B	Class A (iii)
I	0.020	0.020	0.006	0.016
II	0.016	0.016	0.006	0.006
III a	0.008	0.016	none	0.006
III b	0.008	0.016	none	none
IV	none	none	none	none

B . . . . oil-filled apparatus. In British practice oil-filled apparatus is allowed smaller clearances between flanges than air-filled apparatus because arcing beneath the oil surface can produce hydrogen-containing gases in the vapor space above the oil, rendering it more hazardous than the comparable air-filled chamber.

It is to be noted that in the United Kingdom no housings are approved for Group IV, the hydrogen, acetylene, carbon disulfide class. The experimentally determined safe gaps for hydrogen were approximately 0.004 in., and the experimenters were unable to determine a gap small enough to be safe for acetylene. British authorities have to date felt that 0.004-in. gaps are too small to be considered practicable for the majority of apparatus. Housings have been approved in the United States for Group A or B service. Most, but not all, have been small housing with threaded joints only. Housings have been approved in Germany for hydrogen service. However, approvals in both countries are always based on individual test. Gap design values are not specified, as they are for other materials.

Mechanical Design Requirements of BS 229

The reader is cautioned that reference should be made to the latest issue of the official British Standard. The material is presented below only as an indication of the philosophy and general requirements of the British approach to flame-proof enclosures.

Enclosures must be of substantial metallic construction, and except for windows there must be no gaskets in the flame path.

Contrary to American practice, however, openings in the enclosure wall may be closed by insulating materials which carry feed-through terminals. Gaps in flanged joints, of course, must meet the requirements set forth in Table 6-2. Warning nameplates must be used indicating that the case must not be opened until after all power has been disconnected, etc. The case must be designed to withstand hydrostatic test pressures of 1.5 times maximum pressure observed under explosion testing, or 50 psi—whichever is greater. Bolt holes shall be not less than $\frac{3}{8}$ in. from the edge of a joint. Bolts must be shrouded, i.e., they must be protected such that they can be removed only by use of a special wrench. This is typical of European practice and is one of the stumbling blocks for standard-ization of explosion-proof enclosure practice throughout the world. In Germany special bolt heads are specified in addition to shrouding.

Comparison of United Kingdom (European) and United States (American) Practice

United Kingdom practice allows considerably larger gaps for a given flange width than would be permitted in an explosion-proof housing for use in this country or Canada. In the United Kingdom a bolt hole is not considered to be a part of the flame path. Bolt shrouding is required, while in the U.S. and Canada common bolts may be used. The most striking difference between British Standard 229 and UL Publication 698 is that in the British Standard, as in most British standards, the reasons for the requirements are given, wherever possible, so that the designer has a rational basis for considering the design requirements.

INSTALLATION OF EXPLOSION-PROOF HOUSINGS

The following material, while generally applicable to any situation, is based primarily on the provisions of the National Electrical Code.

Because of the possibility of pressure piling, and because of the possibility of communication of a hazard from one location to another through conduit, it is required that seals be used in all conduit entering enclosures containing arcing or high-temperature devices, in all conduit leaving Division 1 and 2 areas, and in all conduit 2-in. trade size or larger entering junction boxes with splices or terminals.

There shall be no union, coupling, box, or fitting in the conduit between the sealing fitting and the point at which the conduit leaves a Division 1 area and enters the Division 2 area, or leaves a Division 2 area and enters a nonhazardous area. Conduit must be installed to prevent water accumulation. Other than those items noted, above no particular installation techniques are necessary beyond those practiced for any enclosure.

MAINTENANCE OF EXPLOSION-PROOF ENCLOSURES

All maintenance or servicing of electrical equipment in explosion-proof enclosures must be done only after the equipment is deenergized. Obviously, the cover of an explosion-proof case must be removed to provide access to electrical equipment for troubleshooting; protection is immediately lost. The practical alternative is, of course, to determine with a combustible gas indicator that the atmosphere in the area is not hazardous if it is necessary to troubleshoot the equipment with power on. In either case extreme caution must be exercised to ensure that the electrical enclosure is tightly closed with all bolts in place and tightened after work is completed.

Because protection offered by an explosion-proof case depends upon cooling of the hot gas by close-spaced flanges or threads, it is imperative that the integrity of flanged joints or threads be maintained throughout the life of the housing. Because permissible gap widths are only a few thousandths of an inch, any foreign material or flange damage can seriously alter the effective gap width. The following precautions, therefore, are simply reasonable considerations in view of the nature of the explosion-proof housing:

a. During assembly or disassembly of the covers the flange surfaces must be treated with great respect. Tools must not come in contact with the flange surfaces. Flanges must not be handled roughly or placed on rough surfaces which will scratch or mar the joint. The covers and cases should always be stored with the flange joints mated to prevent accidental damage to the flange surfaces.

b. Cleanliness must be observed in order that foreign materials will not be trapped between the flanges, enlarging the gap beyond a safe dimension. While an explosion-proof enclosure is in service it is not easy for foreign material to enter the gap. However, in the process of disassembling a cover the material may be picked up on the joints. After disassembly of a cover the joints should be cleaned carefully, removing old grease, dirt, paint, or other material from the joints, if necessary using a solvent such as kerosene. If necessary, the joints should be lubricated before they are reassembled. Sensible precautions must be exercised to prevent a lubricated joint from picking up dirt before it is reassembled. Similar precautions for cleanliness and care in disassembly must be exercised with threaded joints. Bearings provided to permit operation of a shaft through the wall of the housing pose no particular problem, although occasionally they will require cleaning and relubrication. Obviously, under no conditions must diametral clearance be increased.

c. In many locations the corrosion of threaded covers and flanges, rotating shafts, bearings, and other operating parts is a serious problem. Metals compatible with the specific corrosive atmosphere should be specified. The use of corrosion inhibitors or lubricants will often slow down the corrosion process. If and when corrosion does occur and corrosion products cannot be removed with solvent, then the explosion-proof case should be considered to have lost its utility. In corrosive locations, it is important that, when a cover is removed, dislodgment of corrosion products does not enlarge the gap. Very often a flanged or threaded joint may corrode appreciably without affecting the gap width until the joint is disturbed when disassembled; the joint on reassembly with clean surfaces may no longer maintain a safe gap width. The walls of an enclosure should be inspected periodically if severe corrosion is anticipated to ensure that they are not weakened by corrosion.

Few, if any, explosion-proof housings are vapor-tight. Under conditions of high humidity, air laden with water vapor will enter the case. A subsequent drop in temperature may condense water within the case. Even if the temperature rises, the water may not evaporate and leave the case before additional water vapor enters the case. Another cooling cycle will condense more water. Eventually a considerable amount of water will accumulate in the bottom of the case. This water must be drained periodically to prevent damage to electrical equipment. Suitable explosion-proof drains are available from many sources.

REFERENCES

1. Underwriters' Laboratories, Inc., Standards for Safety No. 698, "Industrial Control Equipment for Use in Hazardous Locations," 6th Edition, December 1949.
2. National Electrical Code, Articles 500 ff.
3. Canadian Standards Association, Standard C130-1963, "Explosion-Proof Enclosures for Electrical Equipment."
4. British Standard 229:1957: "Flameproof Enclosure of Electrical Apparatus."
5. Phillips, H., "A Reaction Rate Theory for Flameproof Enclosures," IEE Paper No. 3902M, IEE Conference Report Series No. 3.
6. "A Review of Electrical Research and Testing with regard to Flameproof Enclosure and Intrinsic Safety of Electrical Apparatus and Circuits," Ministry of Fuel and Power, 1943, London.
7. Matson, E. F., R. E. DuFour, and W. C. Westerberg, "An Investigation of Large Electric Motors and Generators of the Explosion-Proof Type For Hazardous Locations, Class I, Group D," Bulletin of Research No. 46, Underwriters' Laboratories, Inc., September 1951.
8. British Symposium on Flameproofing and Intrinsic Safety, 1962, IEE Conference Report Series No. 3, Discussion, p. 59.
9. Lewis, B., and G. Von Elbe, "Combustion Flames and Explosions of Gases," 2nd Edition, Chapter VIII, Academic Press, New York, 1961.
10. Kisselstein, C. F., "Explosion-Proof Enclosures; Design, Tests, and Maintenance," Proceedings of 1960 Symposium on Safety for Electrical Instrumentation in Hazardous Areas," ISA, Pittsburgh.

Chapter 7

Reduction of Hazard by Purging

The use of purging to reduce hazard is recognized in Article 500-1 of the National Electrical Code: "In some cases, hazards may be reduced or hazardous areas limited or eliminated by adequate positive-pressure ventilation from a source of clean air in conjunction with effective safeguards against ventilation failure. It is recommended that the authority enforcing this Code be consulted before such layouts are prepared."

In the 1962 revision of the National Electrical Code, paragraph 501-8 further recognizes use of purging in a more specific manner: "501-8 (a) Class I, Division 1. In Class I, Division 1 locations, motors, generators, and other rotating machinery shall be (1) approved for Class I locations (explosion-proof), or (2) of the totally enclosed type supplied with positive-pressure ventilation from a source of clean air with discharge to a safe area, so arranged to prevent energizing of the machine until ventilation has been established and the enclosure has been purged with at least ten (10) volumes of air, and also arranged to automatically de-energize the equipment when the air supply fails, or (3) of the totally enclosed inert-gas-filled type supplied with a suitable reliable source of inert gas for pressuring the enclosure, with devices provided to ensure a positive pressure in the enclosure and arranged to automatically de-energize the equipment when the gas supply fails. Totally enclosed motors of types (2) or (3) shall have no external surface with an operating temperature in °C in excess of eighty percent (80°) of the ignition temperature of the gas or vapor involved, as determined by ASTM test procedure (Designation: D-286-30). Appropriate devices shall also be provided to detect any increase in temperature of the motor beyond design limits and automatically de-energize the equipment. Auxiliary equipment shall be of the type approved for the location in which it is installed."

ISA Recommended Practice RP12.4 was first issued in 1960. This Recommended Practice, concerning instrument purging for reduction of hazardous area classification, was prepared in order to remedy the serious lack in the National Electrical Code of a specific recommendation for instrument installations, and to fill a need for a commonly recognized safe practice for the instrument industry.   RP12.4 goes well beyond the general statements of NEC 500-1 to make specific recommendations for instrument purging.   This chapter is largely based on RP12.4, to which the reader is referred for specific requirements.

Before pursuing the specific requirements for purging, it should be noted that the use of purging to reduce hazard or to reduce the classification of a hazardous location is applicable not only to Class I hazards, i.e., hazards due to gases or vapors; purging is also used in Class II locations, to prevent dust accumulation from interfering with proper function of equipment, as well as to increase safety.   If gases or vapors enter an instrument case while the purging system is shut down, reactivation of the purging system will reduce hazard as the flammable material is swept out of the instrument case. Some have argued that if the hazard is a Class II or III hazard caused by dust or flyings, a purge system may increase hazard rather than reduce it. They argue that if the purge system is inoperative for a time and dust or flyings enter the case, reactivation of the purging system may disturb the combustible material which had settled on the floor of the case, suspending it once more in the atmosphere and causing a hazard where prior to the purge none had existed. Others feel that no practical purge system is likely to cause air to flow with sufficient velocity to stir up a dust cloud and maintain the dust in suspension.

Purging techniques can certainly be adopted to reduce the degree of any Class I hazard; they may in fact constitute the only practical method for designing some equipments to be used in Group A or B hazardous locations. It was pointed out in Chapter 6 that the minimum safe gap for Group A and B hazards such as acetylene and hydrogen is so small that for large equipments, at least, it is impractical to consider explosion-proof housings. Relatively few equipments have been certified as explosion-proof for Group A and B hazards, and these have mostly been of small volumes and threaded construction. If equipment must operate at high energy levels and yet must be easily accessible for adjustments or servicing, then oil immersion, hermetic sealing, or other techniques may also not be applicable. Purging, however, can be adapted to any situation.

CLASSIFICATION OF PURGING SYSTEMS

ISA RP12.4 defines three types of purging installations:

Type Z—Purging to reduce the classification within an enclosure from Division 2 to nonhazardous.

Type Y—Purging to reduce the classification within an enclosure from Division 1 to Division 2.

Type X—Purging to reduce the classification within an enclosure from Division 1 to nonhazardous.

The requirements for each type of purging can be rationalized in terms of the philosophy of hazard reduction presented in Chapter 5. Type Z purging, which reduces the area classification within the case from Division 2 to nonhazardous, permits installation of ignition-capable equipment in the purged case. In order to have an explosion, the purge system must fail and there must also be simultaneous process equipment failure. Because two independent failures are required there is no necessity to provide additional safeguards in the purge system. To do so would be analogous to wearing a belt and suspenders—safe, but uneconomical.

Type Y purging reduces the classification of the enclosure from Division 1 to Division 2 and permits the use of nonincendive equipment inside the enclosure. Two independent failures, one in the equipment and one in the purge system, must occur before there can be an explosion, so that no additional safeguard in the purge system is necessary.

Type X purging reduces the classification within the enclosure from Division 1 to nonhazardous and, therefore, permits the use of ignition-capable equipment inside the enclosure. Because the environment outside the enclosure is Division 1 and the equipment within the enclosure may be ignition-capable, failure of the purge system constitutes a single occurrence, which changes the probability of explosion from essentially zero to essentially one. In this case it is therefore necessary to provide an additional safeguard in the purging system. An interlock must be provided so that the equipment within the enclosure will not be operative unless the purge system is functioning. Accidental opening of the enclosure while a hazardous atmosphere exists around it must also be prevented.

GENERAL REQUIREMENTS FOR ALL TYPES OF PURGING

Protection by means of purging requires that the purging system prevent flammable material outside the enclosure from entering the enclosure by maintaining a small positive pressure differential between the inside of the enclosure and the outside. It is essential therefore that the enclosure to be purged be of robust physical construction so that accidents of foreseeable nature and the conditions of use will not damage the enclosure to an extent that the purge system is unable to maintain the required positive pressure differential. Windows must be $\frac{1}{4}$-in. thick tempered glass, shatterproof glass, or other shatterproof material suitable for its environment and conditions of use.

The recommendations adopted by ISA in RP12.4 are intended only for application to instrument cases and similar enclosures. Maximum internal volume of the cases covered by RP12.4 is 10 ft^3. The ratio of the maximum internal dimension to the minimum shall not exceed 10:1. This figure is consistent with instrument case construction practice. The recommendations may not be specifically applicable to enclosures designed to a larger ratio. If a case were constructed so that the ratio of the maximum internal dimension to the minimum exceeeded 10:1, depending upon the location and size of vents in the case, it would not necessarily be safe to assume that a single inlet of purging gas would adequately maintain the case free of combustibles. This assumption is, however, justified for case proportions in common use.

If a case contains an auxiliary enclosure, or is connected to one, the auxiliary enclosure may either be purged as though it were separate or it may be considered to be a part of the main case. In the latter instance, the auxiliary enclosure must be connected with the main case by vents top and bottom, each to be of an area at least 1 in.^{2} per 400 in.^{3} of volume.

The source of purging medium is specified only to the extent of defining requirements that any prudent individual would feel to be reasonable. The purge supply obviously should be clean, free of dust or liquids which might impair the operation of the equipment in the enclosure, and should certainly be free of flammable vapors, which would defeat the purpose of purging. Instrument quality compressed air is considered an acceptable purging gas. Plant air is usually not clean enough to be satisfactory purging medium for instruments. Inert gas may be used.

If air is the purging medium, the air compressor inlet must be located in a nonhazardous area. The entire suction line should preferably be in a nonhazardous area. If this is not practical—for example, if the suction line must pass through the hazardous area in order to reach a nonhazardous area at some height above ground— the suction line must be constructed in order to avoid leaks. Both physical and chemical damage to the suction line must be considered in its design.

SPECIFIC REQUIREMENTS FOR PURGING INSTALLATIONS

Type Z Purging (to Reduce Division 2 to Nonhazardous)

Typical installations for Type Z purging are sketched in Figure 7-1. Note that only an indicator is required to show that the purging system is operative. The probability that a process fault will make the location hazardous before failure of the purge system is noticed is assumed to be nil. Any indicator or alarm, if electrical, must meet the requirements of its location. If pressure devices are used, no valve may be installed between the pressure device and the case. Any restriction between the case and the pressure device shall be no smaller than the smallest restriction on the supply side of the pressure device. This requirement is imposed to minimize the likelihood of plugging.

If the case is to be opened it must either be ascertained first that the area is nonhazardous, or power must be removed from the instrument. If an instrument case has been opened, it must be purged with four case volumes of the purging medium before it is energized again, unless the atmosphere within the case is known to be nonhazardous and 0.1 in. water pressure exists inside the case. An analysis justifying the four-case volume initial purge requirement is given in Appendix A.

When the purging system is in operation it must maintain within the purged enclosure a pressure of at least 0.1 in. of water. The flow required to maintain this pressure is immaterial and is

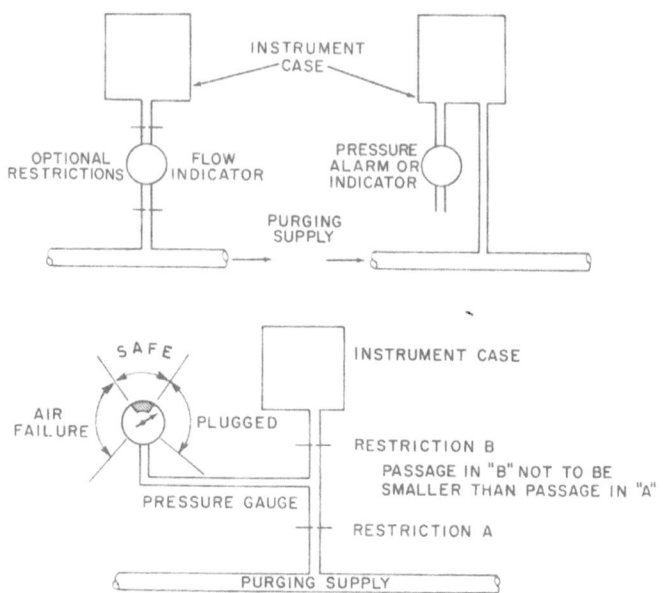

Fig. 7-1. Acceptable installations for Type Z and Y purging (from ISA RP 12.4).

solely a function of the construction of the case. At the time 0.1 in. was selected as the requirement for RP12.4, it was considered by many to be an extraordinarily low pressure. However, the thinking of ISA Committee 8D-RP12 has, in effect, been independently ratified by the International Electrotechnical Commission, whose committee on purging arrived at a recommendation of 0.2 in. of water. A water pressure of 0.1 in. is the static pressure exerted by a 15-mph wind. The purge system will be effective against any wind of lesser velocity than 15 mph. If a purged instrument case were acted upon by a 15-mph wind it is improbable that the atmosphere could be hazardous. A 15-mph wind would so effectively disperse the vapors from any likely source of flammable material that there would be no hazard.

Case temperature of the Type Z purged case shall not exceed 80% of the ignition temperature in °C of the gas or vapor involved when the equipment is operated at 125% of rated voltage.

A red warning nameplate must be placed on the instrument so that it is visible before the case is opened. The nameplate must state that the case shall not be opened unless the area is known to be nonhazardous or unless the power has been removed from the instrument. If any internal surface temperatures may exceed 80% in °C of the ignition temperature of the gas or vapor involved under normal operating conditions at 125% of rated voltage, the warning nameplate must also contain a statement that power must be removed for (x) minutes to permit the unit to cool to safe limits before the door is opened, if the area is hazardous. Alternatively, the portion of the equipment with the offending hot spot may be separately housed and separately purged so that the surface temperature of this secondary enclosure is below the stipulated temperature. This secondary enclosure must then bear a warning nameplate stating that its cover may not be removed for (x) minutes to permit the unit to cool to a safe temperature.

Type Y Purging (Division 1 to Division 2)

No interlocks are required for Type Y purging because an explosion could only occur after failure of the purge and failure of the equipment within the purged enclosure.

Type Y purging must meet all the requirements of Type Z purging previously described. However, because the instrument case is located in a Division 1 area and there is a high probability that a flammable mixture surrounds it, certain additional safeguards are required.

Equipment mounted within the enclosure shall be nonincendive, i.e., it shall conform to the requirements for a Division 2 location (See Chapter 9). The unit shall be fused so that in the event of a short circuit within the case, release of 20% of the available energy will not burn through the case or raise the external surface temperature to 80% of the ignition temperature in °C of the gas or vapor involved. This requirement recognizes that even though the purge system is capable of removing all flammable material from the enclosure, failure of wiring within the enclosure can cause an arc at the enclosure wall. The resulting hot spot might ignite flammable vapors or gases external to the enclosure. In order to provide a safeguard against this occurrence, therefore, the relationship between the maximum fuse size, case thickness, and the gas or vapor expected outside the enclosure is given by the nomograph in Figure 7-2. This nomograph is based on computations made by J. A. Clark and J. A. Beutler, and reported in the Proceedings of

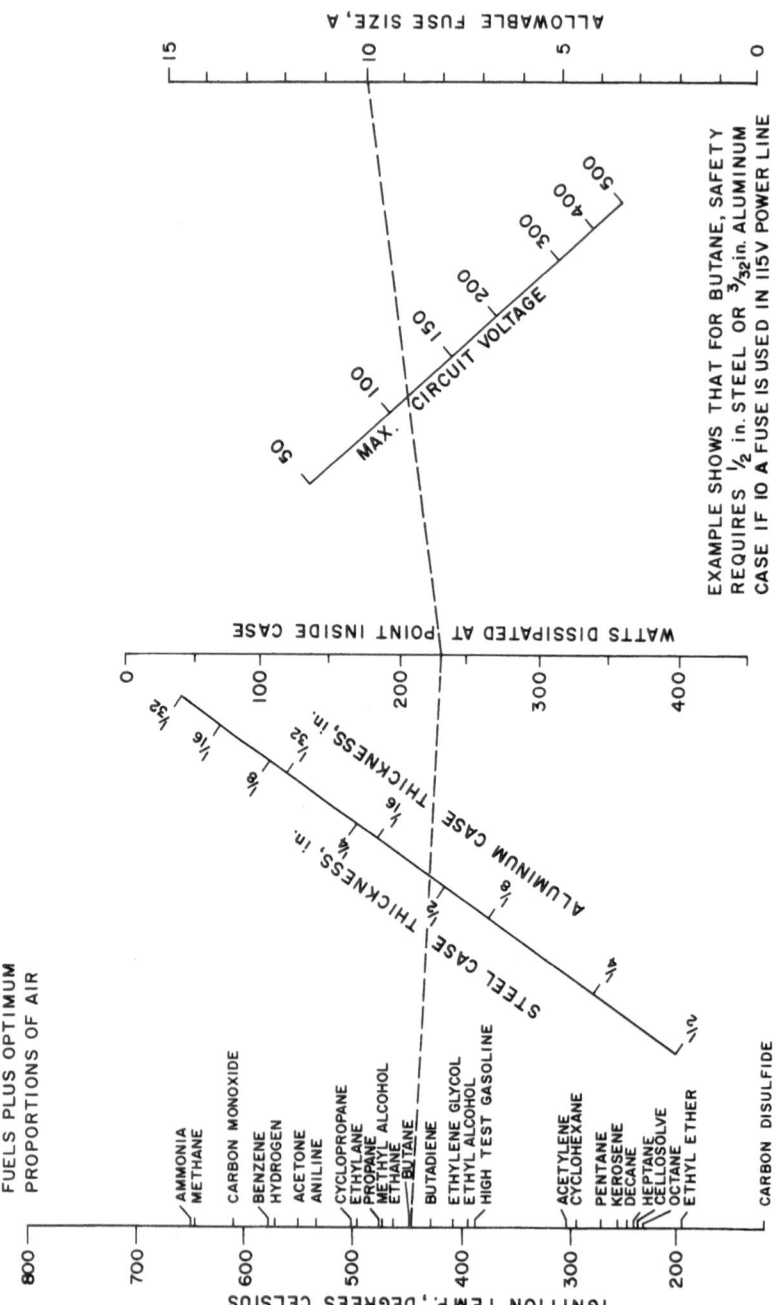

Fig. 7-2. Case thickness, fuse size (from ISA RP 12.4).

the ISA Symposium on Safety for Electrical Instrumentation in Hazardous Areas, Wilmington, Delaware, February 3, 1960. If a double-wall construction, or box-within-a-box construction, is used, and if the purge is connected to the inside box to purge both boxes, fuse size for circuits within the inner box may be increased by a factor of 10. The minimum spacing between the two walls must be at least 10 times the wall thickness.

Type X Purging (Division 1 to Nonhazardous)

Type X purging, because the purging installation is designed to permit the operation of ignition-capable equipment within an enclosure located in an area where the atmosphere is presumed to be frequently flammable, is by far the most critical of purging

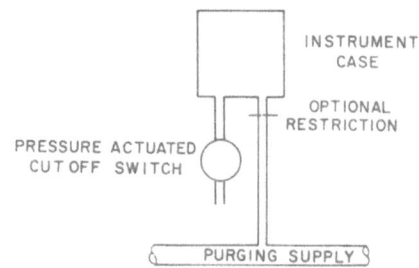

PREFERRED ARRANGEMENT

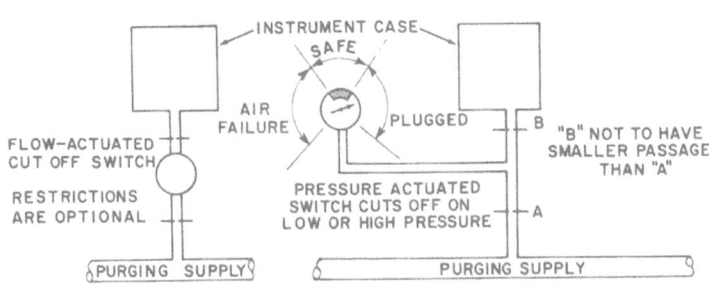

ALTERNATE ARRANGEMENTS

Fig. 7-3. Type X purging layouts (from ISA RP 12.4).

situations. Because the purge is the only safeguard, the purging system must be designed so that its failure automatically removes power from the equipment. This meets the requirement of Chapter 5 that two independent occurrences be required to change the probability of an explosion from 0 to 1. In this case the two independent occurrences are failure of the interlock system and failure of the purge.

All of the requirements for Type Z and Y purging must be met. This especially includes hot spot limitations, case thickness and fuse size, and pressure switch installation requirements. In addition, a device must be incorporated to automatically remove potential from all circuits within the enclosure which are not suitable for Division 1 locations if the purging supply fails. This cutoff switch may be pressure-actuated or flow-actuated. It must be suitable for Division 1 even though it is located within the instrument case, since it may be energized before purging has removed all flammable gas from the case. Another requirement stemming directly from the fact that the atmosphere around the case is presumed to be hazardous a high percentage of the time is that unless tools or a key are required to open the enclosure, the door must be provided with an automatic disconnect switch. The switch must be suitable for Division 1 locations.

A timing device must be incorporated to prevent power from being applied until after a length of time sufficient to allow four case volumes of purged gas to pass through the instrument case while maintaining an internal case pressure of at least 0.1 in. of water. The timing device must meet the requirements of its location (Division 1, even if inside the case).

As with other types of purging, a nameplate must be prominently displayed which warns against opening the case unless the area is nonhazardous, or unless power has been removed, and which states that power shall not be restored until the case has been purged for (x) minutes.

APPENDIX A: DERIVATION OF INITIAL PURGE VOLUME REQUIREMENT

Consider a case of total volume V_T divided into n compartments of equal volume with communicating passages so that all partial volumes are in series:

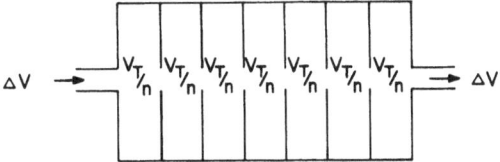

If the concentration of combustible material (gas or vapor) in the first compartment is C_1 and a volume of purge gas, ΔV, of combustibles concentration C_P is introduced, assuming perfect mixing in the first volume (this will be assumed for subsequent sections also), the resulting change in concentration in the first chamber, ΔC_1, is

$$\Delta C_1 = \frac{C_1 V_T/n + C_P \Delta V}{V_T/n + \Delta V} - C_1$$

In differential form,

$$\frac{dC_1}{dV} = \frac{-(C_1 - C_P)}{V_T/n}$$

Using the Laplacian operator method and defining C_{10} as the concentration in chamber 1 before any purge gas is added,

$$SC_1(s) - C_{10} + \frac{C_1(s)}{V_T/n} = \frac{C_P}{SV_T/n}$$

$$C_1(s) = \frac{C_P + S(V_T/n)C_{10}}{[S(V_T/n) + 1]S}$$

For the second section the purging input will be volume ΔV with concentration C_1, and

$$C_2(s) = \frac{C_1(s) + (V_T/n)C_{20}}{(S + n/V_T)V_T/n}$$

where C_{20} is initial concentration.

$$C_2(s) = \frac{C_P + S(V_T/n)C_{10} + S(V_T/n)[(V_T/n)S + 1]C_{20}}{S[(V_T/n)S + 1]^2}$$

after substituting the expression for $C_1(s)$.

The concentration in the Mth and last section, the one of interest in determining the amount of purge volume required, is

$$C_n(s) = \frac{C_P + S(V_T/n)C_{20}[(V_T/n)S + 1] + \ldots + S(V_T/n)[(V_T/n)S + 1]^{n-1}C_{no}}{S([V_T/n]S + 1)^n}$$

For the usual situation the concentration of combustible gas or vapor can reasonably be assumed to be sensibly uniform throughout the case so that $C_{10} = C_{20} = C_{30} = C_{no}$ and

$$C_n(s) = \frac{C_P + S(V_T/n)C_{10}\{1 + [(V_T/n)S + 1] + [(V_T/n)S + 1]^2 + \ldots [(V_T/n)S + 1]^{n-1}\}}{S[(V_T/n)S + 1]^n}$$

Solving this equation and transforming back to the original variables C_n, the concentration of combustible in the nth section, and V, the total volume of purge gas, the general solution is

$$C_n = C_P + (C_{10} - C_P)E^{-nV/V_T}\left[\sum_{k=0}^{k=n-1} \frac{1}{k!}\left(\frac{nV}{V_T}\right)^k\right]$$

If the purge air is clean, as it should be, $C_P = 0$, and the concentration as a function of purge volume for specific numbers of sections of equal volume is given by

$$C_1 = C_{10}E^{-V/V_T}$$

$$C_2 = C_{10}E^{-2V/V_T}\left[1 + \frac{2V}{V_T}\right]$$

$$C_3 = C_{10}E^{-3V/V_T}\left[1 + \frac{3V}{V_T} + \frac{1}{2}\left(\frac{3V}{V_T}\right)^2\right]$$

$$C_4 = C_{10}E^{-4V/V_T}\left[1 + \frac{4V}{V_T} + \frac{1}{2}\left(\frac{4V}{V_T}\right)^2 + \frac{1}{6}\left(\frac{4V}{V_T}\right)^3\right]$$

$$C_5 = C_{10}E^{-5V/V_T}\left[1 + \frac{5V}{V_T} + \frac{1}{2}\left(\frac{5V}{V_T}\right)^2 + \frac{1}{6}\left(\frac{5V}{V_T}\right)^3 + \frac{1}{24}\left(\frac{5V}{V_T}\right)^4\right]$$

The curves in Figure A-1 show the concentration in the last section in terms of the initial concentration C_{10}, plotted against total purge volume relative to total case volume V_T. Even in the worst case, that of a single undivided volume, four volumes of purge air will reduce the concentration to less than 2% of the initial value.

The lowest L.E.L.'s listed in NFPA pamphlet No. 325 are about

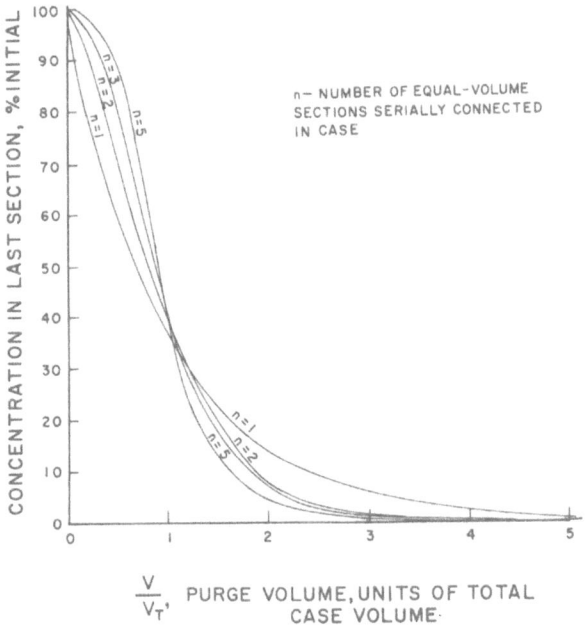

Fig. A-1. Effectiveness of purge.

0.6%. Four volumes of purge are therefore adequate even when the initial concentration of such vapors is at a ridiculously high level of 30%. Any subdivision of the case into serially connected volumes improves the effectiveness of the purge.

Since the requirement for initial purge of four case volumes is safe for even a single section case, it follows that any subdivision, even when the subdivisions are of unequal size, is in the direction of improving purge effectiveness.

REFERENCES

1. RP12.4, "Instrument Purging For Reduction of Hazardous Area Classification," Instrument Society of America, Pittsburgh.
2. McCarron, R., "Considerations in Instrument Case Purging," Proceedings of 1960 Symposium on Safety for Electrical Instrumentation in Hazardous Areas.
3. Beutler, J.A., and J.A. Clark, "Heat Transfer and Computational Considerations in the Design of Instrument Cases for Operation in Hazardous Atmospheres," Proceedings of 1960 Symposium on Safety for Electrical Instrumentation in Hazardous Areas, Instrument Society of America, Pittsburgh.

used in a Division 1 area to make equipment nonincendive, in order to permit Type Y purging rather than the more complex Type X purging installation. However, except in a Group A or B hazardous location, if the equipment cannot be made intrinsically safe one could just as well use an explosion-proof housing without oil immersion. The need for accessibility for calibration and maintenance of instruments makes oil immersion unattractive for most devices.

In Division 2 locations it is possible that oil immersion can be used to render equipment nonincendive, but it is more likely that sealing or encapsulation or, in large assemblies, purging, will be used.

SEALING

The principle of sealing, commonly but unnecessarily called "hermetic" sealing, is recognized in the National Electrical Code, paragraph 501-3 (b) (1). This paragraph states that general-purpose enclosures may be used in Division 2 locations if make-break contacts are hermetically sealed against the entrance of gases or vapors. However, there is no definition in the National Electrical Code nor is there a definition formalized and issued by Underwriters' Laboratories stating what constitutes a hermetic seal. Since there exists no standard test or definition issued by those responsible for the Code, approval of a specific hermetically sealed device is left to the discretion of the Code-enforcing authority who has no criteria other than his own experience and judgment upon which to rely.

If one were to apply literally the dictionary definition of a hermetic seal, very few devices could meet the requirements. The dictionary definition of a hermetic seal is one which is "made perfectly closed or air-tight so that no gas or spirit can enter or escape." In practice, of course, any seal does pass gas or vapor to some extent. In the limit even the metallic or glass container itself is somewhat permeable to vapors and gases. In practice, therefore, a hermetic seal is simply a controlled leak. Military specifications define several leak rates which determine the class of hermetic seals. In specification MIL S-8484 seals are defined as Grade A if they do not leak at a rate greater than 1 std cm^3 of air/year/inch of seal at a differential of one atmosphere. Grades B and C seals, respectively, leak at rates less than 99 and 9,999

std cm^3 of air/year/inch of seal per atmospheric pressure differential. A Grade D seal is defined as one which leaks in excess
of 10,000 std cm^3 of air/year/inch of seal per atmospheric pressure
differential. MIL S-6106 specifies for many types of relays a
leakage rate not exceeding 1μ-ft^3/hr. This is approximately 300
cm^3/yr.

A comprehensive testing program, including many types of
seals, was carried out in 1954 by Bedwell and Meyer. Their
results show that seals obtained by silver soldering, or even
aluminum soldering, remained Grade A even after having been
subjected to 100% relative humidity at 25°C for 30 days; 270 min.
of vibration in the range of 10-55 cycles at 0.060 in. total excursion;
and three temperature cycles from -65 to 200°C. The welded joints
tested were of quite variable quality and demonstrated the need for
special training to obtain good seals. Test of a variety of adhesive
type seals showed, as one might expect, great variation in ability
to seal, but many were consistently of Grade C or better quality.
Generally, O-rings with rectangular grooves or natural rubber
gaskets with rectangular grooves gave very good seals, i.e., a very
large percentage of those tried were Grade A. However, in general,
composition type seals utilizing cork and asbestos did not seal
successfully and gave a high percentage of Grade D seals. Metal-to-
metal seals utilizing thin copper or lead gaskets on 90° ridges gave
good results. The copper gaskets resulted in 96% of the seals tested
being Grade A; the performance of lead gaskets was more variable.
Tests of lapped surfaces gave scattered results. It seems reasonable that most commercial seals which make a serious attempt to
exclude the external atmosphere are probably very close to Grade C
or better under industrial conditions, which are seldom as severe as
the conditions of these tests.

In order to give the reader a better feel for what the grades
noted above imply in mechanical construction, the following table
lists the hole size which for one atmospheric pressure differential
across a 0.030-in. wall would give a leak rate corresponding to the
various grades of seal. These hole diameters are calculated from
the equation

$$Q = 8.97 \cdot 10^{16} \frac{r^4}{l} (P_2^2 - P_1^2)$$

where Q is the leak rate in standard cubic centimeters/year/inch/
atmosphere; r is the radius of hole (inches); l is the hole length

Grade	Leak rate	Hole dia. (in.)
A	<1 cc/y/in./atm	$48 \cdot 10^{-6}$
B	<99 cc/y/in./atm	$152 \cdot 10^{-6}$
C	<9999 cc/y/in./atm	$498 \cdot 10^{-6}$
D	>9999 cc/y/in./atm	$> 498 \cdot 10^{-6}$

(inches); and P_1, P_2 are the pressures on either side of the leak (atmospheres).

In connection with the use of hermetic seals it is often suggested that high internal pressures be used as a means of rendering a system safe. However, in the industrial application of hermetically sealed devices, pressurization alone is of no significant value in increasing safety.

Most commercial hermetically sealed devices, if pressurized at all, do not have initial internal pressure greater than 1.2 atm, absolute. This internal pressure in a typical relay would drop to 1.1 atm in a year or so if the seal were Grade A. A Grade C seal would allow the pressure to drop from 1.2 to 1.1 atm in an hour or so. Even if initial pressurization were at 2 atm, a Grade C seal would allow the pressure to drop to 1.1 atm in $2\frac{1}{2}$ hr. In the preceding examples an end point of 1.1 atm was chosen because it is sufficient internal pressure to guarantee that barometric pressure changes and pressure changes caused by a diurnal temperature cycling would not cause internal pressure to become less than the external pressure. Reversal of pressure differential would cause pumping through the seal. Since the useful life of industrial equipment is far longer than that of the safe period using even a Grade A seal, it is obvious that pressurization alone is not sufficient. Even if a seal in a metallic container were initially so perfect that pressurization would not be lost, a glance at the above table indicates that at almost any time within the lifetime of the equipment corrosion could cause small unnoticeable pinholes and protection would be quickly lost. The basis for the above statements is further discussed in Appendix B-1.

It is quite obvious from the foregoing considerations that hermetic seals have not been accepted as safe because they are pressurized or because they do not leak. It is therefore of more than casual interest to answer the question, "Why is a hermetic seal safe?" The answer is that a hermetic seal is safe when it imparts to the device being protected a time response much longer than the probable duration of a hazardous atmosphere around the device. When this is so, not enough of an external flammable atmosphere is transferred through the seal to raise the inside concentration to a hazardous level. N o t e : There is an essential condition implicit in the above statement which is of paramount importance to the safe application of seals. The a v e r a g e concentration in the atmosphere around sealed devices must always be nonhazardous because the concentration inside will eventually reach the average concentration outside the sealed enclosure.

Transport of flammable material across the seal of an enclosure will occur either because of flow caused by pressure drop across the seal, or by diffusion of material through the seal. The following paragraphs will treat of both breathing and diffusion. It will be shown that for any reasonable assumptions, almost any seal which purports to be a seal at all will be adequate from the standpoint of breathing. Diffusion effects, however, determine the quality of seal required for safety.

For consideration of the effects of breathing, assume the limiting case of a seal which offers absolutely no impediment to flow of gas in and out of the enclosure but does prevent wind and convection currents from causing an interchange of internal and external atmosphere.

Assume that there exists a 6-in. Hg daily cycling of pressure drop across the seal, caused by ambient temperature and barometric pressure changes. This is an extreme assumption. In New York during the period 1885 to 1958 the t o t a l r a n g e of barometric pressure was 2.63 in. Hg. To have a 6 in. Hg variation, it is necessary to assume that to this barometric pressure change is added the effect of a 60°F daily temperature change.

Assume that a 10% hydrogen atmosphere exists outside the enclosure. During the half of the day when the pressure outside the enclosure is higher than that inside by the assumed 6 in. Hg, the mass of gas inside the enclosure will be increased 20% by the addition of outside atmosphere. If the initial concentration inside the enclosure were 0, then the new concentration will be 1.67% hydrogen $(10 \cdot 0.2/1.2)$. During the second half-day, when the pressure outside the chamber drops below that inside, the mass returns to the initial value. The concentration, however, remains the same. On the second day, additional inflow will raise the concentration to 3.06%, which is still below the lower explosive limit of hydrogen.

To achieve a flammable mixture inside the enclosure we must assume a completely ridiculous combination of circumstances. We must assume a more severe daily cycling pressure differential across the seal than would ever exist in practice; we must assume 10% hydrogen existing outside the instrument for a period greater than 24 hr. If we assume 5% hydrogen, the atmosphere would have to be present for more than 4 days before the 4% LEL could be reached inside the enclosure. The efficacy of the seal, therefore, lies in its long time constant compared to any probable duration of the hazard external to it. Breathing of a real seal is treated in more detail in Appendix B-2.

From the above considerations, it can be concluded that breathing determines the quality required of the seal only to the extent that the seal must prevent convection and windage from transporting flammable material. How leaky a seal may be is determined by diffusion effects which are considered in the following paragraphs.

The fundamental equation for diffusion is

$$dQ = - \Delta \; \frac{dc}{dx} \; dydz$$

where dQ is the amount of material passing through an area $dydz$ in the direction of x in a time dt; dc/dx is the rate of increase of concentration in the direction of x; Δ is the coefficient of diffusion.

For considering diffusion through a hole in an enclosure the equation can be written in the form

$$\frac{dC_i}{dt} = \Delta \frac{C_0 - C_i}{V_0 L} \frac{\pi d^2}{4}$$

where V_0 = volume of enclosure (cm^3); C_i = concentration inside enclosure; C_0 = concentration outside enclosure; L = enclosure wall thickness (cm); d = diameter of hole in enclosure (cm); Δ = diffusion coefficient, (cm^2/sec). Solving this differential equation for t, the time to reach concentration C_i, we obtain

$$t = \frac{4 V_0 L}{\Delta \pi d^2} \ln \frac{C_0 - C_{i0}}{C_0 - C_i}$$

where C_{i_0} is the initial concentration inside the enclosure. In the usual case C_{i_0} is near zero.

It can be seen that for a given hole diameter the most severe case will be when the enclosure volume is small.

Assume $V_0 = 8$ cm^3, typical of a small relay; $L = 0.075$ cm; $d = 2 \cdot 10^{-3}$ cm (Grade D seal); $C_{i_0} = 0$; $C_l = 4\%$, LEL of hydrogen; $C_0 = 10\%$; $\Delta = 0.65$, typical of hydrogen;

$$t = \frac{(4)\,(8)\,(0.075)}{0.65\,\pi\,(1)\,(2 \cdot 10^{-3})^2}\,\ln\frac{10}{10-4} = 1.7 \cdot 10^5 \text{ sec} = 48 \text{ hr}$$

If the outside concentration were 5%, the time for diffusion to raise the inside of the enclosure to the LEL would be 153 hr. These calculations show that even if a small volume and a highly mobile gas are assumed, diffusion effects are small enough that most sealing means would give effective protection as long as the average concentration outside the enclosure is below the LEL.

It can be concluded from the above consideration of breathing and diffusion that to meet the intent and spirit of paragraph 501-3(b) (1) of the NEC, "hermetic" seals are not required. All that is required is an effective seal which need not be as good as Grade C.

That a Division 2 location where the National Electrical Code permits hermetic seals to be used is on the average nonhazardous is easily accepted. That most Division 1 locations are also on the average nonhazardous may not be so obvious.

It cannot be proved with statistics that in Division 1 areas also the atmosphere outside closed systems or containers is not above the lower explosive limit for long periods of time. Data are just not available. However, the following arguments support this assumption.

1. If the atmospheric concentration of the flammable material were above the LEL for extended periods of time, it is likely that possible ignition by the electrical equipment would be an academic matter entirely. Ignition by sparks from tools, shoe nails, lightning, or electrostatic discharges would almost certainly destroy the plant even if there were no electrical equipment within it.

2. Although not all flammable materials are toxic, most are either toxic or discomforting. Most materials are toxic or cause discomfort at concentrations of less than 0.1%, much lower than the LEL.

3. Except in closed rooms or closed process vessels gas or vapor hazards tend to be self-dispersing. The cost of product loss required to maintain a continuous supply of flammable material would not go unnoticed.

The above rationale explains why the use of "hermetic" seals has long been permitted in Division 2 areas in spite of the fact that there are no standards and specifications for "hermetically sealed" equipment. Because present area classification procedures may assign a Division 1 classification to an area whether it is above the LEL 100% of the time as in a processing vessel, or a very small percentage of the time as in the usual instrument installation, it is not possible to recommend the use of "hermetic" seals unrestrictedly in Division 1 locations. A seal obviously cannot be used in a location where the average concentration is above the LEL. The concentration inside the sealed device attempts to reach the average level of concentration outside of the enclosure. If this average level is below the LEL, an installation with sealed ignition sources will be safe whether the location is classified Division 1 or Division 2. If the average concentration is above the LEL the installation will be unsafe. A distinction between Division 1 areas where the average concentration is above the LEL and those where the average concentration is below the LEL is not now recognized in the United States. However, some European classifications designate an area which is for all practical purposes always hazardous (above the LEL) as Division 0.

REQUIREMENTS FOR SEALED DEVICES

A distinction must be made between what is likely to be considered acceptable by the Code-enforcing authority at the present time and what is really needed in a seal for a Division 2 area. On the basis of the foregoing consideration of breathing and diffusion, the only requirement of an effective seal from a safety standpoint is that the enclosure have structural integrity with regard to its intended environment, that its surface temperature be less than 80% of the ignition temperature of the gas or vapor being considered, and that whatever seal design is used causes the time constant of the enclosure to be on the order of several hours. Construction must also be such that the seal is not destroyed by normal maintenance procedures.

Although it is undoubtedly true that most gasketed constructions or even most metal-to-metal joints will adequately meet all of these requirements, until there is a Recommended Practice for effective seals which recognizes all these factors, it is likely that most Code-enforcing authorities will require soldered joints, although essentially equivalent sealing methods, such as adhesive joints, may sometimes be accepted.

ENCAPSULATION OR POTTING

For the purpose of this book, encapsulation or potting is considered to be any embedment of a component or assembly in a solid medium such as plastic, ceramic, tar, etc. There may or may not be an additional enclosure surrounding the solid medium. Tars and waxes used for potting or encapsulating transformers have customarily been used inside a supporting can. However, many devices are now potted or encapsulated using epoxies, PVC, or other plastics which do not require additional support.

The application of potting or encapsulation techniques to reduction of hazard can be justified on the basis of either one of two methods of protection which have already been considered in detail. Because the potting material quite effectively seals the ignition source from the surrounding atmosphere, the potted device can be considered safe because the potting acts as an effective seal. If the voids within the encapsulated assembly are small, the assembly might also be considered safe because it is explosion-proof. That explosion pressure would not rupture the encapsulant if ignition occurs in a void would have to be demonstrated by test.

One of the certain uses of encapsulation will be in intrinsically safe circuits where it is necessary to guarantee that a particular junction point in the circuit cannot be grounded or connected to some other point of a circuit. Encapsulation of such a junction with appropriate concern for mechanical strength and compatibility with the surrounding environment can reduce to zero the probability that the encapsulated joint is electrically accessible.

There are no recognized requirements for encapsulation for safety purposes. It is likely that ISA will prepare a Recommended Practice. However, common sense dictates that the encapsulation must be designed so that the completed assembly is compatible with its environment. The encapsulant must have such strength and such mechanical design that it will not crack or fracture as a result of thermal or mechanical shock it would receive in foreseeable usage. It must be chemically stable with respect to any gases or vapors to which it would be exposed. It must, of course, be capable of withstanding all the environmental conditions to which it will be exposed. The temperature of any point normally accessible to the combustible atmosphere must be below 80% of the ignition temperature in °C of that atmosphere.

The application of encapsulated assemblies will undoubtedly grow. Because encapsulation offers protection equivalent to that of a hermetic seal, such an approach has already been accepted and will continue to be accepted without serious question in Division 2 areas, although at the present time there is no explicit basis in the National Electrical Code for permitting such construction.

APPENDIX B-1: DERIVATION OF AN EQUATION FOR LOSS OF PRESSURE IN A SEALED SYSTEM

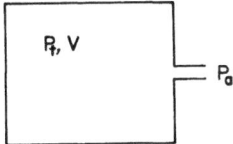

P_t is the pressure inside system (atm); V is the system volume (cm^3); P_a is the pressure outside the system (atm); l is the seal length (in.); P_{to} is the initial system pressure (atm); K is the leak rate (cc/yr/in./atm^2); and t is the time (yr).

$$- Kl(P_t^2 - P_a^2) = \frac{V}{P_a} \frac{dP_t}{dt}$$

The left-hand side of this equation is the conventional equation for flow through a small restriction, taking density changes into account (See Bedwell and Meyer). The right-hand side of the equation is the change in volume of gas in the system referred to pressure P_a.

This equation has the solution

$$P_t = \frac{P_a(1 + C_2 \epsilon^{-2P_a^2\,(Kl/V)t})}{(1 - C_2 \epsilon^{-2P_a^2\,(Kl/V)t})}$$

at

$$t = 0, \; P_t = P_{to}$$

Therefore,

$$C_2 = \frac{P_{to} - P_a}{P_{to} + P_a}$$

So

$$P_t = P_a \left[\frac{P_{to} + P_a + (P_{to} - P_a) \, \epsilon^{-2P_a^2 \,(Kl/V)t}}{P_{to} + P_a - (P_{to} - P_a) \, \epsilon^{-2P_a^2 \,(Kl/V)t}} \right]$$

Solving for t in the above equation,

$$t = \frac{V}{2P_a^2 \, Kl} \ln \frac{\left(\dfrac{P_t}{P_a} + 1\right)\left(\dfrac{P_{to}}{P_a} - 1\right)}{\left(\dfrac{P_t}{P_a} - 1\right)\left(\dfrac{P_{to}}{P_a} + 1\right)}$$

If t is in days and V is in cubic inches,

$$t = \frac{2985}{P_a^2} \frac{V}{Kl} \ln \frac{\left(\dfrac{P_t}{P_a} + 1\right)\left(\dfrac{P_{to}}{P_a} - 1\right)}{\left(\dfrac{P_t}{P_a} - 1\right)\left(\dfrac{P_{to}}{P_a} + 1\right)}$$

In typical hermetically sealed devices V/l is in the range 0.2 to 10 in.^{3}/in.

If P_t is taken to be 1.1 and P_a is taken to be 1.0, for the extremes of the V/l range,

$$t = \frac{597}{K} \ln \frac{2.1}{0.1} \frac{P_{to} - 1}{P_{to} + 1} \quad \text{or} \quad t = \frac{29850}{K} \ln 21 \frac{P_{to} - 1}{P_{to} + 1}$$

If seal is Grade A and $K = 1$ and initial pressure P_{to} is 2 atm,

$$t = 1160 \text{ days} \qquad \qquad t = 58{,}200 \text{ days}$$
$$= 3.18 \text{ yr} \qquad \text{or} \qquad = 159 \text{ yr}$$

If seal is Grade C, $K = 10^4$ and $P_{to} = 2$ atm,

$$t = 2.8 \text{ hr} \qquad \qquad \text{or} \qquad \qquad 5.82 \text{ days}$$

APPENDIX B-2: DERIVATION OF EXPRESSIONS FOR SEAL BREATHING

We first derive the equation for half-day flow through a seal caused by ambient temperature and barometric pressure variations.

For a small restriction the flow equation is

$$Q = \frac{Kl}{365}(P_2^2 - P_1^2)$$

where Q is flow rate (cc/day); K is leak rating (cc/yr/in. of seal/atm); l is length of seal; and P_2 and P_1 are pressures on opposite sides of seal (atm).

If P_2 and P_1 are near 1 atm this expression can be simplified by replacing $(P_2^2 - P_1^2)$ by $2(P_2 - P_1)$ or $2\Delta P$, to get

$$Q = \frac{Kl}{182.5}(P_2 - P_1) = \frac{Kl}{182.5}\Delta P$$

For considering breathing of a seal, we use the following model:

P_2 is the pressure inside the system (atm); P_1 is the pressure outside the system (atm); A is the fractional change in internal pressure caused by ambient temperature changes; B is the fractional change in external pressure; V_0 is the system volume (cc); V is the volume of gas flow in or out of the system; and $\phi = 2\pi d$, where d is in days.

$$P_2 = P_{20} - \frac{P_{20}}{V_0}\int Q\,d\phi + AP_{20}\sin\phi$$

$$P_1 = P_{10} - BP_{10}\sin\phi$$

Note that it is assumed that A and B are acting in the direction to simultaneously increase or decrease the pressure drop across the seal. This is a very conservative assumption.

Assuming that P_{20} and P_{10}, the initial values of P_2 and P_1, are both 1 atm, and noting that

$$V = \int Q\,d\phi \quad \text{and} \quad Q = \frac{dV}{d\phi}$$

the flow equation can be written as

$$\frac{182.5}{Kl}\frac{dV}{d\phi} + \frac{V}{V_0} = (A + B)\sin\phi$$

The solution to this equation is

$$V = \frac{(A + B)}{1 + \left(\dfrac{Kl}{182.5\,V_0}\right)}\frac{Kl}{182.5}\left[\frac{Kl}{182.5\,V_0}\sin\phi - \cos\phi + \epsilon^{-\frac{Kl\phi}{182.5\,V_0}}\right]$$

For a practical range of variables the exponential term can be neglected. This expression can be written

$$V = \frac{(A + B)}{\left[1 + \left(\dfrac{Kl}{182.5\,V_0}\right)^2\right]^{1/2}}\frac{Kl}{182.5}\cos(\phi + \theta)$$

where $\theta = \operatorname{Arctan} Kl/182.5\,V_0$.

The maximum flow volume during the day will be when $\cos(\phi + \theta) = 1$:

$$V_{max} = \frac{(A + B)}{\left[1 + \left(\dfrac{Kl}{182.5\,V_0}\right)^2\right]^{1/2}}\frac{Kl}{182.5}$$

$$= \frac{(A + B)\,V_0}{\left[1 + \left(\dfrac{182.5\,V_0}{Kl}\right)^2\right]^{1/2}}$$

If $K \to \infty$ then $V_{max} = (A + B)V_0$, as used in the illustration in the text.

Having calculated the half-day flow for a given system, we are now in a position to determine how long it will take for the concentration inside the system to reach a specified concentration, if the outside concentration is specified.

C_0 is the concentration outside system; C_i is the concentration inside system; C_{i_0} is the initial concentration inside system; d is the time in days.

The development of the required equation can be carried out by recording the amount of contaminant material in the system after V volumes are breathed in and the resulting concentration in the system before breathing out. After breathing out, the concentration in the system of course remains the same, but the amount is decreased.

Amount of Contaminant in System after Breathing in	Concentration Before Breathing Out

Initially

$$C_{10} V_0 \qquad\qquad C_{10}$$

1st cycle

$$C_{10} V_0 + C_0 V \qquad\qquad \frac{C_{10} V_0 + C_0 V}{V + V_0}$$

2nd cycle

$$\frac{C_{10} V_0^2 + C_0 V V_0}{V + V_0} + C_0 V \qquad\qquad \frac{C_0 V}{V + V_0} + \frac{C_{10} V_0^2 + C_0 V V_0}{(V + V_0)^2}$$

3rd cycle

$$\frac{C_0 V V_0}{V + V_0} + \frac{C_{10} V_0^3 + C_0 V V_0^2}{(V + V_0)^2} + C_0 V \qquad \frac{C_0 V}{V + V_0} + \frac{C_0 V V_0}{(V + V_0)^2} + \frac{C_{10} V_0^3 + C_0 V V_0^2}{(V + V_0)^3}$$

At the end of the portion of a cycle during which volume flows into the system,

$$C_i = C_{io} \left(\frac{V_0}{V + V_0}\right)^d + C_0 \frac{V}{V_0} \left[\frac{V}{V + V_0} + \left(\frac{V_0}{V + V_0}\right)^2 + \left(\frac{V_0}{V + V_0}\right)^3 + \cdots \left(\frac{V_0}{V + V_0}\right)^d\right]$$

The expression in the brackets is of the form

$$\gamma + \gamma^2 + \gamma^3 + \cdots + \gamma^d$$

The general form is $1 + \gamma + \gamma^2 + \gamma^3 \cdots \gamma^{n-1}$, where

$$n = d + 1$$

Σn terms $= [(1 - \gamma^n)/(1 - \gamma)] - 1$, where $\gamma = V_0/(V + V_0)$.

$$C_i = C_{io} \left(\frac{V_0}{V + V_0}\right)^d + C_0 \left[1 - \left(\frac{V_\rho}{V + V_0}\right)^d\right]$$

Solving for d,

$$d = \frac{\ln\left(\frac{C_0 - C_i}{C_0 - C_{io}}\right)}{\ln\left(\frac{V_0}{V + V_0}\right)}$$

REFERENCES

1. Mil-S-8484 (USAF), Seals and Seal Testing Procedure, June 25, 1954.
2. Mil-R-6106c (ASG), Relays, Electric, Aircraft, General Specification for.
3. Bedwell, D. C., and E. A. Meyer, "Leakage Testing of Sealed Electronic Enclosures," Electrical Manufacturing, pp. 127-133, December 1955.
4. Magison, E. C., and L. E. Cuckler, "Reducing the Hazard from Electrical Components and Assemblies by Hermetic Sealing, Encapsulation or Liquid Immersion," 1960 Symposium on Safety for Electrical Instrumentation in Hazardous Areas, Instrument Society of America, Pittsburgh.

Chapter 9

Intrinsically Safe and Nonincendive Systems

INTRINSIC SAFETY

As a result of the efforts of ISA Comittee 8D-RP12 the 1956 edition of the National Electrical Code included for the first time a paragraph recognizing the concept of intrinsic safety. Paragraph 500-1 states, "Equipment and associated wiring approved as intrinsically safe may be installed in any hazardous location for which it is approved, and the provisions of Articles 500–517 need not apply to such installation. Intrinsically safe equipment and wiring is incapable of releasing sufficient electrical energy under normal or abnormal conditions to cause ignition of a specific hazardous atmospheric mixture. Abnormal conditions will include accidental damage to any part of the equipment or wiring, insulation or other failure of electrical components, application of over-voltage, adjustment and maintenance operations, and other similar conditions."

The application of the principle of intrinsic safety to electrical equipment and wiring for use in hazardous locations represents an approach which is quite different from the methods discussed in earlier chapters. In an intrinsically safe system, safety is afforded by the design of the system, not by addition of protective measures to the system. Safety, therefore, exists throughout the life of the equipment, during maintenance, and in spite of maintenance. Safety of the sort obtained by application of explosion-proof housings, on the other hand, is safety which is readily lost as a result of care-lessness. Should a mechanic fail to properly install the cover after a maintenance operation, safety is lost. Safety can also be lost because of corrosion or mechanical damage to the equipment.

It is essential that it be understood that the term "intrinsically safe" applies to circuits or "equipment and wiring," not to devices. In most situations only a part of a system is so energy-limited that it can be classified intrinsically safe. Almost any industrial instrument loop, for example, is somewhere connected to the power line. Quite obviously, the power line is ignition-capable, and not intrinsically safe. Therefore, only a portion of the system is designed to be intrinsically safe. The remainder of the system is designed to be suitable for its location. Most often this latter portion is located in a Division 2 area, but it could be located in a Division 1 area and purged or housed in an explosion-proof case. In either case, the system must be designed to prevent the non-intrinsically safe portion of the system from feeding enough energy to the intrinsically safe portion of the circuit to cause ignition, even under failure conditions.

The first applications of the principles of intrinsic safety were in England, where laboratory work on explosions of flammable gases were started in 1922 at what is now the Safety in Mines Research Establisment. This work resulted first in flameproof enclosure standards. It was later expanded to cover standards for intrinsically safe equipment. Impetus for the effort came from a series of mine disasters, and early applications were in mines. However, the concept of intrinsic safety is now accepted and widely used in other industries in the United Kingdom.

During the 1950's interest in applying and using the principles of intrinsic safety mushroomed in Europe, the Soviet Union, and in the United States. All over the world, increased use of electrical equipment in hazardous locations demanded review and revision of electrical installation practices. This widespread interest resulted in the establishment of a committee to establish an international standard on intrinsic safety under the auspices of the IEC. To date, a standard has not been adopted.

Adoption of intrinsic safety as a working technique in the United States was spearheaded by ISA with the establishment of ISA Committee 8D-RP12 in 1949. In the early years of committee activity progress was quite slow. There was wide divergence of opinion about designing a safe system and equally wide variance in practice in installing a "safe" electrical installation. However, under the chairmanship of F. L. Maltby a great deal of progress has been made. Acceptance of the principle of intrinsic safety in the United

States can be attributed directly to the educational activities of this Committee.

The Committee's goal has been to promote uniform, safe, and economical practices for use of instrumentation in hazardous areas. Probably the single most important decision made by the Committee was that it would prepare Recommended Practices which were both safe and economical, and that they would be based on the application of sound engineering judgment after a thorough consideration of available technical information. These Recommended Practices would contain few, if any, arbitrary rules, and would not be bound by existing practices which could not be justified by a reasonable evaluation of pertinent technical considerations.

Implicit in this position is that if the Recommended Practices are based on thoughtful evaluation of applicable facts they can be used by anyone who has studied and understands the pertinent technical literature. This is a radical departure from the concept of a central approval body, which is accepted everywhere else in the world. Even in the United States there are still many persons who cannot conceive of installing an intrinsically safe system unless a recognized approval body has tested and approved the system.

REQUIREMENTS FOR INTRINSICALLY SAFE INSTALLATIONS

The National Electrical Code states in principle the nature of intrinsically safe equipment and wiring, but the definition gives no hint of the design and constructional features which make equipment and associated wiring intrinsically safe. The material in the following paragraphs is based on ISA Recommended Practice RP12.2. Although specific requirements have, in general, not been published by domestic or foreign approval bodies, it can be started with assurance that the philosophy of ISA is not greatly different from that of these approval bodies. The significant exception is that ISA maintains that approval of a system as intrinsically safe can be made by anyone skilled in the art, as well as by a recognized approval body. This philosophy is not, as it may first appear, really radical. It represents only an extension of present practice in this country regarding matters of safety and design. Though most electrical equipment destined for use by untrained, unskilled users is submitted to U.L. or other testing agencies for approval as meeting their standards for personnel and fire safety, few industrial measurement or control instruments are submitted. The decision that a device will be safe under the conditions of its intended use is made by the user or his insurance underwriter. The installation of thousands of explosion-proof housings each year which have not been approved by U.L. or F.M. is a pertinent example of the exercise of judgment by the user in the absence of formal testing and certification. Such enclosures are safe and are recognized as such because they are designed to meet conservative standards. Some of the specific requirements of RP12.2, of course, may differ significantly from those of an approval body.

The National Electrical Code defines intrinsically safe equipment and wiring as "incapable of releasing sufficient electrical energy under normal or abnormal conditions to cause ignition of a specific hazardous atmospheric mixture." ISA, when preparing RP12.2, had to answer for itself and for the users of RP12.2 the following questions:

1. What level of energy is incapable of igniting the specific hazardous mixture?
2. What is "a specific hazardous atmospheric mixture?"
3. What are normal and abnormal conditions?

These questions have been answered on the basis of the facts concerning electrical ignition presented in Chapters 3 and 4 and the probabilistic philosophy of hazard reduction outlined in Chapter 5. If the probability for underwriting purposes of a circuit igniting a specific atmospheric mixture is reduced to zero, it meets the requirement of an intrinsically safe circuit. In order to make the concept of intrinsic safety useful and economic, the requirements for intrinsically safe systems must eliminate all probable combinations of circumstances which could cause ignition, without being overly conservative.

When confronted with a document such as ISA RP12.2 it is difficult for one to visualize the wide diversity of opinion which existed and still exists in some quarters regarding the interpretation of the National Electrical Code definition. To further elucidate the ISA point of view, as represented by RP12.2, several examples of extreme views which have been rejected by ISA as being unnecessarily and uneconomically conservative are summarized below.

1. "All intrinsically safe equipment must be intrinsically safe for hydrogen atmospheres." This view has found some support in the United States, and is favored by many Europeans. It is certainly a safe approach, although one glance at ignition energy data shows hydrogen to be so much more easily ignited than common gases or vapors, most of which are typified by NEC, Class I, Group C and D materials, that to design all equipment to be intrinsically safe in a hydrogen atmosphere is unnecessarily restrictive and uneconomical.

2. "All possible combinations of failures must be considered in determining whether or not energy levels might rise above a permissible safe level under fault conditions." This statement, though superficially plausible, would eliminate a system from being considered intrinsically safe if any portion of the system were connected to a 120V power line. One could always postulate for any equipment which does not have a self-contained power source, a possible (though not probable) train of failures extending back to an ignition-capable source.

3. "All possible modes of failure must be considered." This too, is a plausible-sounding requirement, but reduced to absurdity this provision would require designing against falling aircraft, runaway trucks, or other calamities of ridiculously remote probability.

GROUND RULES FOR ESTABLISHING THE SPECIFIC REQUIREMENTS OF RP12.2

In the following paragraphs are summarized the most fundamental definitions used as a basis for preparing specific requirements in RP12.2.

Specific Hazardous Atmospheric Mixture

A specific hazardous atmospheric mixture could be of any stated composition at any temperature or pressure. Unless otherwise stated, however, it is considered to be the most easily ignited mixture of the designated vapor or gas with air at normal ambient temperature and atmospheric pressure. Although the concept of intrinsic safety can be applied to devices installed within processing vessels at pressures or temperatures much different from those at normal ambient, these installations do not represent a high percentage of the total. Because most reliable experimental data are limited to measurements at normal temperature and pressure it seemed most prudent to limit RP12.2, at least for the present time, to that area of application where it is most urgently needed and for which the experimental data are also supported by experience. That the inflammable mixture to be considered is the one which is most easily ignited follows directly from the fact that it is impossible to predict in an industrial situation what the concentration of the hazardous atmosphere may be. The most conservative assumption is therefore made. A specific hazardous atmospheric mixture is denoted because there are large differences in ignition energy among gases and vapors. A system which is intrinsically safe for methane whose minimum ignition energy is about 0.25 mJ would not necessarily be safe for hydrogen, whose minimum ignition energy is about 0.02 mJ. Circuitry safe for hydrogen would, of course, be safe for methane.

Normal and Abnormal Conditions

Normal conditions comprise the normal operation of the equipment, including the effects of maximum supply voltage and extreme environmental conditions within the ratings of the equipment. Normal conditions also include opening, shorting, and grounding of all wires connecting enclosures in the intrinsically safe portion of the system. This provision recognizes that in most industrial systems wiring external to devices is selected and installed by the user, and because of its exposed location is very likely to be opened, shorted, or grounded accidentally or deliberately during the useful life of the system. Exceptions to this provision will be few, but might include systems where connecting means are specially designed and installed in protected conditions to render grounds, shorts, and opens so improbable that they can be treated as ordinary failures.

Abnormal conditions include all probable failures of components and wiring. The number of failures to be considered is defined on the basis of the philosophy outlined in Chapter 5, so that in all cases there are the equivalent of two safeguards lying between a safe and an unsafe situation.

Safe Energy Levels

Energy levels which can be permitted in an intrinsically safe system are determined by considering practically realizable modes of ignition. In Chapter 4 it was shown that at voltage levels to be found in typical instrument systems even the most improbable combination of electrode material, speed, and condition—and concentration of hazardous mixture—requires more energy for ignition than the minimum ignition energy measured by the high-voltage capacitance discharge method. Minimum ignition energy determined by that method, therefore, is not necessarily a sensible criterion for permissible energy levels in intrinsically safe systems of low voltage. Energy limits must be established on the basis of the practically obtainable ignition mechanisms that can be foreseen.

SPECIFIC REQUIREMENTS FOR INTRINSICALLY SAFE EQUIPMENT

A. Method of Approval

ISA RP12.2 recognizes two equally valid ways in which equipment and wiring can be approved as intrinsically safe. Either method may be used and either method is equally acceptable.

1. Equipment may be approved as intrinsically safe by approval of the Safety Enforcement Authority with or without ignition testing. The Safety Enforcement Authority may be the plant safety officer, a representative of the underwriter, or a municipal official. Whoever he may be, he holds the final responsibility for approving the installation. He may, in granting his approval, exercise his personal judgment, accept approval by a testing agency, or reach his decision in any other manner he deems suitable.
2. Equipment may be approved as being intrinsically safe without ignition testing if it meets the specific requirements of RP12.2.

The parallel and alternative methods of approving systems are provided because it is not the Committee's intention that RP12.2 run counter to the responsible judgment of recognized approval agencies. However, it is also necessary that RP12.2 provide a mechanism for economical, safe approval of systems as being intrinsically safe.

To provide a mechanism by which systems can be deemed intrinsically safe without the necessity of ignition testing, RP12.2 establishes a set of requirements which in some particulars are more restrictive than might be applied by some approval agencies and which will exclude from approval without test some equipments which are intrinsically safe. These systems may, of course, be approved with or without ignition testing by the Safety Enforcement Authority.

If a system is judged to be intrinsically safe because it meets the stipulated requirements of RP12.2, ignition testing is not only unnecessary, it is a senseless waste of effort. The requirements of RP12.2 allow a sizable additional safety factor (4:1 on current and voltage levels) over the reference test data to allow for measurement errors or unknown factors when a particular design is being evaluated. From a safety standpoint the current and voltage levels permitted by the reference curves are already "safe" by a large factor. They represent levels at which ignition would occur less than once in at least 100 trials, when an improbably favorable combination of most easily ignited concentration of the flammable material, electrode geometry, and speed are used.

There are many safe circuits which cannot be approved without testing by applying the standards of RP12.2 because present knowledge is not sufficient to allow safe current and voltage levels to be stated as a function of component or circuit characteristics. The most common examples are circuits with iron-core inductors. All existing reference curves are based on air-core inductors. Iron-core inductors may be significantly less efficient in transferring energy to the arc because of losses within the core. An iron-core inductor, therefore, may sometimes be safe at considerably higher current levels than an air-core inductance of the same nominal value. It is not possible today to predict from electrical constants the relative incendivity of an iron-core inductor compared to an air-core inductor. Therefore, until either a feasible method of calculation or more empirical data become available, the safety of circuits with iron-core inductors must be demonstrated by actual ignition testing if the current levels are above those permitted for air-core inductors. There is a similar situation when coils operate in magnet structures with soft-iron pole pieces.

B.   Requirements for Approval Without Testing

The principal requirement of RP12.2 for approval of a device as intrinsically safe without ignition testing is that current and voltage levels in any portion of the circuit must not exceed a safe value.

RP12.2 includes reference curves relating current in inductive circuits and voltage in capacitive circuits to the value of inductance and capacitance. These curves are based on actual ignition data for the gases specified under conditions so much more severe than would be encountered in an industrial installation that safety is assured.

If a device has no normally operating contacts, it is required that under normal conditions, including opens, grounding, or shorting of external connections, as described previously, the current or voltage must not be greater than 25% of the values determined from the reference curves. Under abnormal conditions, i.e., under failure situations, no two faults in combination shall cause the current or voltage to rise above 50% of the level from the reference curve.

If a circuit contains a normally operating contact, under normal conditions or under fault conditions, the currents and voltages in the circuit must not exceed 25% of those determined from the reference curves. For the purposes of RP12.2 a contact which is designed to operate is assumed to be a normally operating contact. A high-limit contact is "normally operating" although it might never actually function during the life of the equipment.

In addition to the limits imposed on current and voltage levels to restrict the energy level in the circuit to safe values, it is also required that no surface temperature in the equipment exceed 80% of the ignition temperature in °C of the specific gas or vapor. It is recognized that small surfaces, such as a straight fine wire, may exceed this temperature limit and not be a source of ignition, but safety of such constructions must be demonstrated by test.

No fuse or circuit breaker shall be considered to limit the currents and voltages to the value stipulated by the reference curves. Limited experimental evidence indicates that ignition can occur while a fuse is blowing. Not enough is now known to specify a practicable, safe manner of selecting a protective fuse, if such exists. All circuit analysis must therefore assume that fuses and circuit breakers do not function.

BASIS FOR THE REFERENCE CURRENT AND VOLTAGE CURVES

Because RP12.2 provides that intrinsically safe equipment and wiring can be approved on the basis of examination, calculation and measurement, the Committee was not constrained to relate the reference curve values to the characteristics of any particular testing apparatus. All British data, of course, are related to the break-spark apparatus or to the intermittent break apparatus. German regulations are related to the PTB slotted disc and counter-rotating brush apparatus. Because the Committee was not constrained to recommend a particular apparatus for testing, it could review all the data on ignition which were available to it and decide which data would serve as the best basis for an American Recommended Practice on intrinsic safety. If one compares the reference curves included in this chapter, which are taken from ISA RP12.2, to the curves of similiar nature in Chapter 4, one sees that

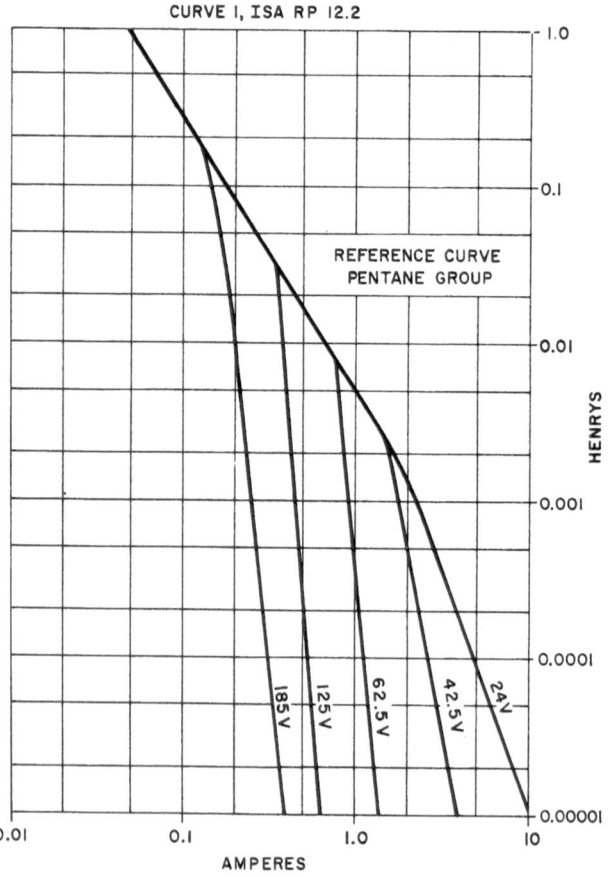

Fig. 9-1. Sample reference curve.

Figure 9-1 for inductive and resistive circuits is drawn on the basis of data taken using the British break-spark and intermittent break apparatus. Comparison of the reference curves for capacitive circuits in Figures 9-4 and 9-6 with Figure 4-10a shows that the zero current curves are similar to the PTB ignition data. Freed from dependence on a particular apparatus, the Committee could select reference levels of a safe, but not overly conservative nature.

In the case of capacitive ignition data there was no serious problem in deciding to utilize German data. These and what little other data were available agreed rather well. However, this was not the case when the Committee decided to use the British data on inductive and resistive circuits as the basis for the reference curves. German data derived from the PTB apparatus were available and were considered to be reliable. However, there were important differences in current levels in the German and English data. Referring to Figure 4-12 in Chapter 4, one can see that there is a difference in ignition current level on the order of 2 to 1, with the German levels being lower at a given inductance. This disparity is not as serious as it appears, however, because the Germans propose to use an additional safety factor of only 1.5; at 0.1 H a circuit could be approved for methane if the current in it were 65 mA or less. The British would approve a circuit of 0.1 H inductance at 95 mA after applying a safety factor of 2. For a circuit of 1.0 H the approvals would be given at 20 and 25 mA, respectively.

In circuits of lower inductance, however, the disparity between published British data and published German data approaches 10 to 1 in current. (See Figure 4-14c). The choice between German and British data in this case cannot be rationalized by considering the difference in size of an additional safety factor. Selection of one level has important implications to the applicability of the concept of intrinsic safety in practical systems. If the German data for methane ignition were to be accepted as a reference, even with the application of an additional safety factor of 1.5, a 50 V system would be limited to a maximum current of 0.33 A under normal conditions. With a safety factor of 2 the British would permit 1.5 A in the same circuit.

The British data were selected for use as reference data for RP12.2 on the basis of the following considerations:

a. The German data were obtained using a tungsten wire operating against a cadmium surface. Figure 4-13 shows that cadmium electrodes cause ignition at lower current levels than steel or platinum electrodes by a factor of 3–4 at low inductance levels. Use of a cadmium electrode therefore heavily biased the PTB data. In the opinion of Committee 8D–RP12, it is not reasonable to establish intrinsic safety criteria on the basis of ignition data obtained using materials not representative of those normally used in instrument construction.

b. Use of British data is indicated on the basis that ignition data were derived using an electrode system giving ignition at the same levels as copper and steel electrodes, which are common instrument construction materials.

c. Safe application of the British data in approving intrinsically safe systems for over three decades attests to the safety and reasonableness of the British standard.

Hot-wire ignition was not a factor in establishing the reference current levels. The committee concluded, after reviewing available data on hot-wire ignition, that hot-wire ignition need not be considered unless there is a real probability that a wire could attain a temperature above 80% of the ignition temperature of the gas or vapor. Even then, unless the wire is coiled to concentrate heat, or is of high-melting-point material such as iron, nickel, nichrome, platinum, or tungsten, consideration of hot-wire ignition will not change the limiting currents determined from break-spark data. Straight copper wire will not cause ignition at currents less than the fusing current. Even for 42-gauge wire, the ignition current for a typical vapor is 4 A, a higher value than could normally be determined from break-spark considerations.

DERIVATION OF REFERENCE CURVES

In RP12.2 reference curves are given for three groups of materials, called "Pentane," "Ethylene," and "Hydrogen" groups. Table 9-1 lists the materials included in each of the groups. The table also shows the classification given in British Standard 1259 for the materials. Although the classifications are almost identical, and the names "Pentane Group," "Ethylene Group," and "Hydrogen Group" are similar to wording on British certificates

TABLE 9-1. Classification of Atmospheric Mixtures of Vapors and Gases

BS 1259 class	ISA RP12.2 group	Gas or vapor	
1	Pentane	Methane (firedamp)	petroleum
2a	—	Ammonia	naphtha
2b	—	(reserved for future allocation)	kerosene

2c	Pentane	(i) HYDROCARBONS	(ii) COMPOUNDS CONTAINING OXYGEN

Alkanes

methane (industrial)
ethane
propane
butane
pentane
hexane
heptane
nonane
cyclobutane
cyclohexane
methylcyclohexane
decahydronaphthalene

Benzenoids

benzene
toluene
xylene
ethylbenzene
trimethylbenzene
naphthalene

Alkenes

butene
cyclohexane
styrene

Mixed Hydrocarbons

turpentine
coal tar naphtha

Oxides (incl. ethers)

carbon monoxide
methoxyethanol
ethoxyethanol
ethyldigol
butyldigol
dibutyl ether

Alcohols and Phenols

methanol
ethanol
propanol
butanol
pentanol
hexanol
octanol
nononol
cyclohexanol
methylcyclohexanol
diacetone alcohol
phenol
cresol

Aldehydes

formaldehyde
acetaldehyde
octaldehyde
paraformaldehyde
paraldehyde
metaldehyde
benzaldehyde

BS 1259 class	ISA RP12.2 group	Gas or vapor	

2c (cont'd.)   Pentane (cont'd.)

Ketones

acetone
ethyl methyl ketone
propyl methyl ketone
butyl methyl ketone
amyl methyl ketone
acetylacetone
cyclohexanone

Esters

methyl formate
ethyl formate
methyl acetate
ethyl acetate
butyl acetate
amyl acetate
methyl acetoacetate
diethyl oxalate

(iii) COMPOUNDS
CONTAINING HALOGENS

Compounds Without
    Oxygen
chloromethane
chloroethane
bromoethane
chloropropane
chlorobutane
bromobutane
dichloroethane
dichloropropane
chlorobenzene
benzyl chloride
dichlorobenzene
allyl chloride

dichloroethylene

Compounds with
    oxygen

acetyl chloride
chloroethanol

(iv) COMPOUNDS
CONTAINING NITROGEN

Amines

methylamine
dimethylamine
trimethylamine
diethylamine
triethylamine
propylamine
butylamine
cyclohexylamine
ethanolamine
diethylaminoethanol
diaminoethane
aniline
dimethylaniline
amphetamine
toluidine
pyridine

Amides

formdimethylamide

Nitro-compounds

nitromethane
nitroethane
nitrobenzene

BS 1259 class	ISA RP12.2 group	Gas or vapor	
2d	Ethylene	(i) HYDROCARBONS cyclopropane ethylene butadiene	(iii) COMPOUNDS CONTAINING NITROGEN acrylonitrile isopropylnitrate
		(ii) OXIDES (incl. ethers and heterocyclics) dimethyl ether ethyl methyl ether diethyl ether dipropyl ether ethylene oxide epoxypropane dioxolane trioxan dioxan tetrahydrofuran tetrahydrofurfuryl alcohol	
2e	Hydrogen	hydrogen blue water gas town gas (coal gas) coke—oven gas	
2f	Unclassified Hydrogen	carbon disulfide acetylene	

of intrinsic safety, the similarity is in the interest of common terminology, and not indicative of a blind adoption of the British classification. As RP12.2 neared completion, the committee decided to use the British list in modified form because it was more inclusive than any other available. However, before the classification was adopted, the placing of materials in subclasses was checked against the other data available to the committee.

The basis for drawing the reference curves for "Pentane Group" materials (Figures 9-1 and 9-4) has already been described. Though

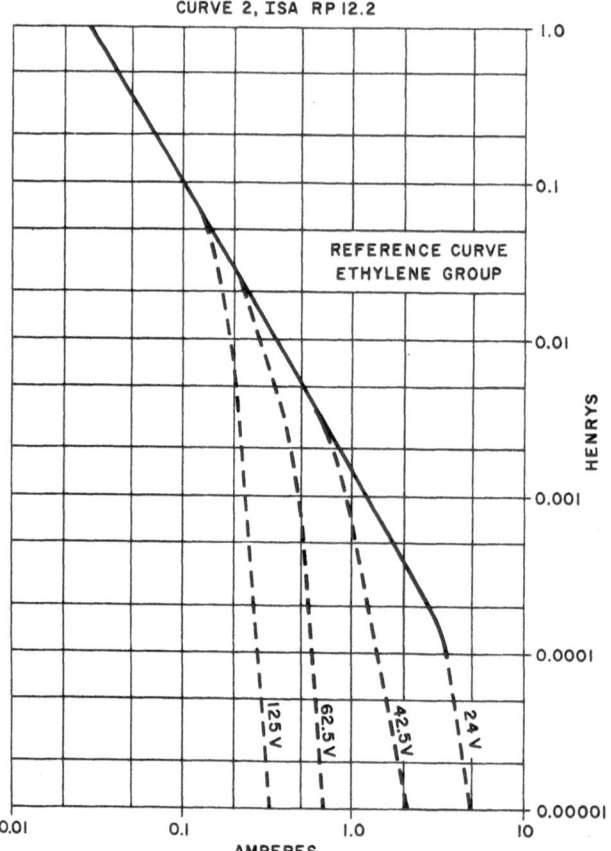

Fig. 9-2. Sample reference curve.

reference to Table 4-8a shows that there are significant differences in break-spark igniting current for materials within the group, these differences are small compared to the additional factor of safety of 4:1 required by RP12.2.

Although published data on ignition of methane gave a firm basis for drawing the "Pentane Group" reference curves, preparation of curves for the "Hydrogen Group" and the "Ethylene Group" required assumptions to be made. Figure 9-3, L-I-V relations for hydrogen, is based on break-spark data at 24 V reported in Electrical Research Association Report G/T259. The higher voltage lines have been drawn in assuming similarity to the methane curve, using voltage relationships reported in VDEO170/0171d2:65, the West German regulation for intrinsic safety.

Figure 9-2 for the "Ethylene Group" is also based on British data, ERA Report D/T106. Curves for voltages other than 24 V were drawn on the basis of assumed similarity to methane ignition, in the absence of empirical data.

In Figures 9-4 and 9-6, the zero current capacitance–voltage relationships are derived from the German data. In Figure 9-5 for "Ethylene Group" materials, the zero current curves were interpolated between the hydrogen and methane curves. Though the

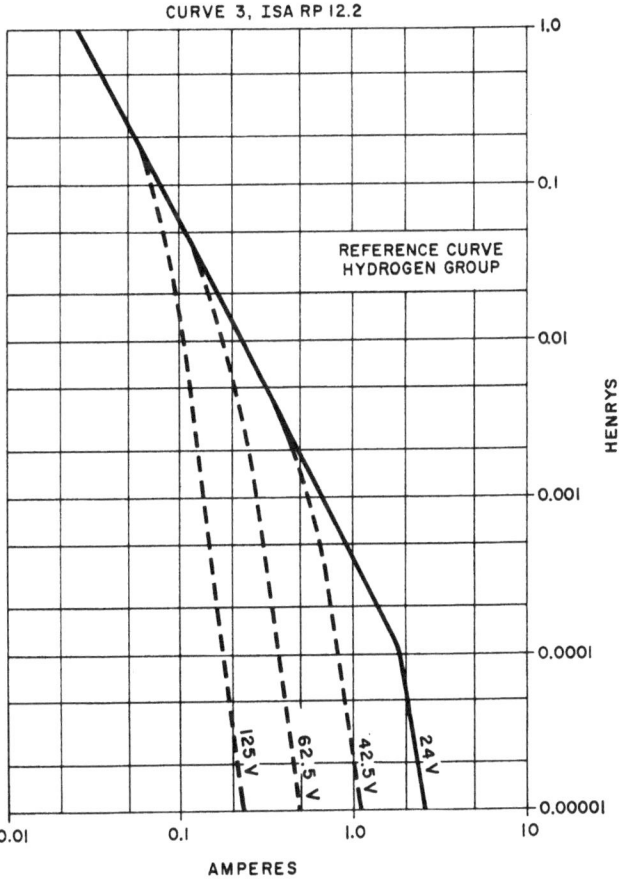

Fig. 9-3. Sample reference curve.

ignition voltages at the same capacitance level for methane and hydrogen are not in the relationship one would predict from the minimum ignition energies of the two materials, it is assumed that it is reasonable to interpolate between the actual data for hydrogen and methane to obtain an ethylene curve using the minimum ignition energies of the three materials as a reference.

On Curves 9-4, 9-5, and 9-6, the relationship between current and voltage at the lowest level of capacitance shown is the same relationship as the voltage–current relationships on Figures 9-1, 9-2, and 9-3 for the lowest inductance. This equality assumes that

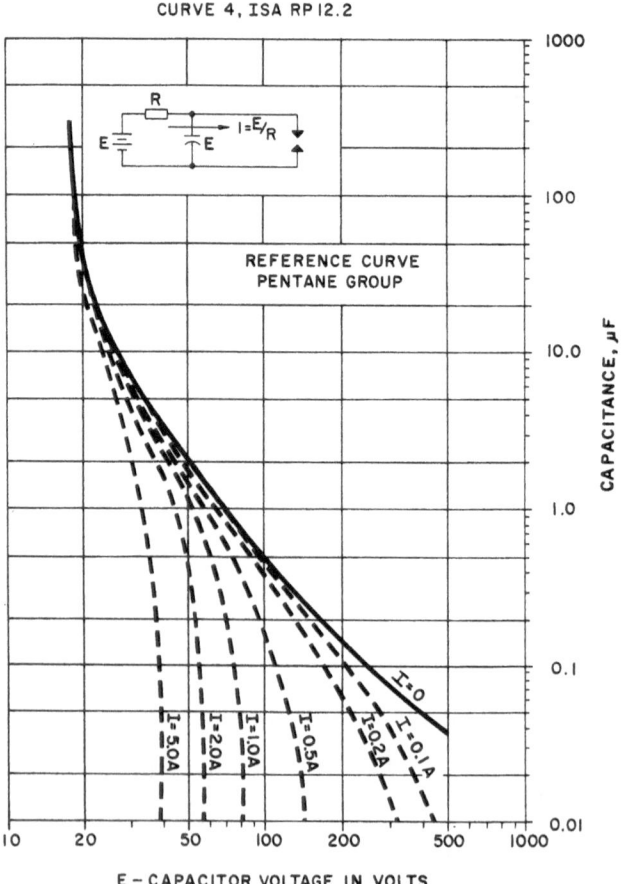

Fig. 9-4. Sample reference curve.

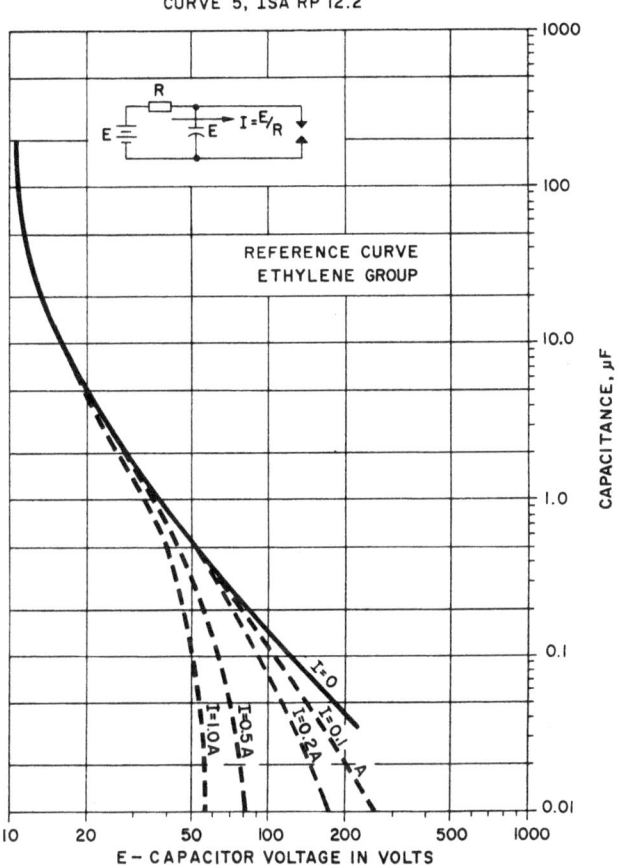

Fig. 9-5. Sample reference curve.

the current required to cause ignition in essentially resistive circuits is the same whether the contacts are closing or opening. The committee felt that to assume this equality for closing contacts is a conservative position, because quenching effects are most likely to require even higher currents with closing contacts.

The relationship between capacitance and voltage for circuit current levels other than zero is calculated using the zero current capacitance and "near-zero capacitance" current data points as fixed points for a given voltage. The calculation was made assuming that the energy contributed by discharging the capacitor and energy

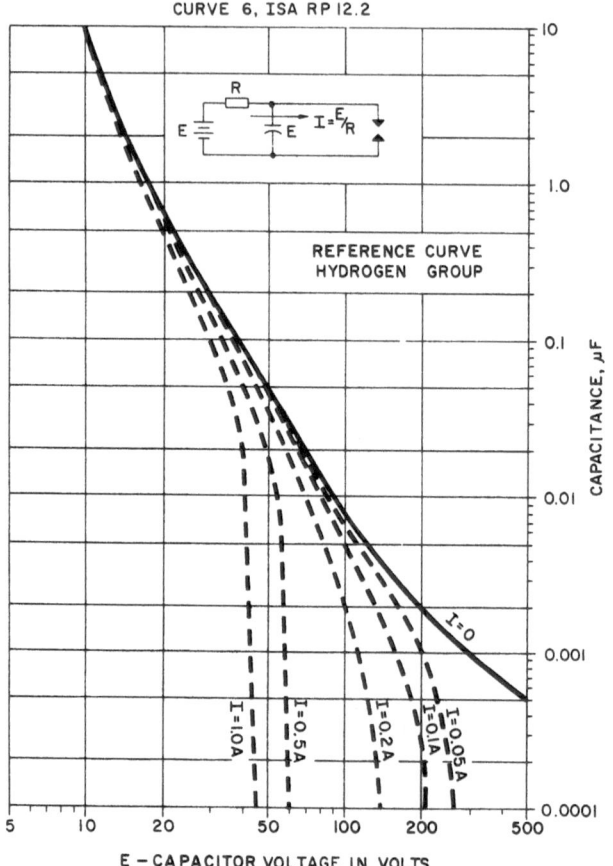

Fig. 9-6. Sample reference curve.

contributed by the short-circuit current are additive, probably a very conservative assumption. For a particular voltage and short-circuit current, the allowable capacitance C was computed from

$$C = \frac{I_{sc} - I}{I_{sc}} C_0$$

where I_{sc} is the "zero capacitance" current required to cause ignition at that voltage; I is the short-circuit current; C_0 is the "zero current" capacitance required to cause ignition at that voltage.

CONSIDERATION OF SAFETY FACTORS

In RP12.2, a 4-to-1 additional factor of safety is applied to the reference data under normal conditions when approval without test is desired.   This allows for uncertainty in knowing circuit constants, errors in measurement, and other such factors.   The factor of 4 might better be called an "ignorance" factor.   The reference levels are already almost ridiculously safe in that they presume a combination of events, i.e., well maintained contacts, optimum speed, and optimum composition of mixture, to occur simultaneously in an improbable fashion.

Under fault conditions, the additional factor of safety is reduced to 2 to 1.   Ignition at reference current and voltage levels is of very low probability.   There is extremely low probability of two independent faults occurring in combination.   These two facts together make application of a higher additional safety factor than 2 to 1 completely unnecessary.

A larger additional factor of safety is applied to circuits containing normally operating contacts purely on the basis of simple prudence. Even though equipment having no contacts and equipment which has an infrequently operating contact may in actuality have essentially the same probability of causing ignition, RP12.2, for simplicity's sake, treats any device which has a contact as though the contact operates frequently.   It was the Committee's feeling that sufficiently few intrinsically safe devices are likely to have normally operating contacts, that lack of a fine distinction in terms of operating frequency would not be a serious restriction to widespread utilization of intrinsic safety.

It is important to recognize that RP12.2 stipulates additional factors of safety of 4:1 under normal conditions, and 2:1 under abnormal conditions only for systems being approved without test.   If the system is tested, such a large factor is not required. The Safety Enforcement Authority may determine the factor to be used. In the United Kingdom, the factor is normally 1.5 to 2. In Germany, the factor is 1.5.

ABNORMAL OR FAULT CONDITIONS

A fault is considered to include opening, shorting, or grounding of any electrical conductor or component, including resistors, capacitors, vacuum tubes, diodes, transistors, etc.—or insulation breakdown in any portion of the circuit—which may affect the available energy in the intrinsically safe portion of the circuit. However, this statement does not imply that all possible connections and all possible failures must be considered. For example, possible shorts between two insulated conductors which are separated by a suitable barrier or which are secured in place so that the conductors are not normally touching need not be considered. One can justify this on the basis of the fact that failure of the barrier or tie-down means plus two independent insulation failures are required to cause a short, and that, therefore, the possibility is too remote to be considered.

The requirement that no two faults in combination shall cause currents or voltages to exceed the levels specified is excepted if one of the required faults is a fault of a "highly reliable" component. A "highly reliable" component is one which because of its design, construction, and installation has essentially zero probability of failing in a way which would raise the current or voltage in the portion of the circuit being evaluated. A good example is a single-layer wirewound resistor constructed on a ceramic mandrel and so mounted that the leads cannot be shorted. Such a resistor can be constructed to have essentially zero probability of failing in a way which reduces its resistance. Therefore, if such a resistor is used to limit current, a drop in resistance which allows current to increase can be presumed to be of zero probability.

NONINCENDIVE EQUIPMENT AND WIRING

A very significant contribution of RP12.2 is a definitive description of nonincendive equipment and wiring. Only the name is new; the concept is old. Nonincendive equipment and wiring is equipment and wiring which in its normal operating condition will not ignite a specific hazardous atmospheric mixture. Such equipment has been recognized without specific denomination for some time in paragraph 501-3(b) of the National Electrical Code. In Division 2 areas equipment without make-and-break or sliding contacts and without hot surfaces may be enclosed in general-purpose housings. In paragraph 501-3(b)(2) slidewire contacts in potentiometers used in conjunction with thermocouples are specifically excepted from the prohibition of sliding contacts because of the obviously low energy levels involved.

RP12.2 extends the usefulness of the concept, however, by recognizing that even arcing contacts are safe and meet the spirit of paragraph 501-3(b) if the energy released at the contacts is maintained well below the value required for ignition. A second important contribution of RP12.2 is a definition of what constitutes a make-and-break contact in which energy must be limited.

The requirements of RP12.2 will be a boon to many instrument users and manufacturers who in the past have negotiated the design of equipment to be used in Division 2 areas almost on an individual basis. There has been no accepted definition of what constitutes safe construction. Therefore, there have been costly and confusing differences in design approach in the treatment of calibration adjustments, disconnect switches, etc.

The requirements for nonincendive equipment and wiring can be summarized as follows:

1. Current and voltage levels in any circuit with make–break contacts must be below 25% of the values given in the reference curves unless the contacts are protected by oil immersion, sealing, or other means suitable for installation in Division 2 areas.

2. Plugs, jacks, and switches which are used for corrective maintenance are acceptable regardless of power level. It is assumed that one should determine that the atmosphere is not hazardous before beginning maintenance operations.

3. No surface temperature may be above 80% of the ignition temperature in °C of the specific gas or vapor unless, as in the case of straight fine wires, the construction is shown to be safe by test.

Nonincendive equipment and wiring, therefore, may contain circuits of very high energy, potentially capable of ignition. However, two failures are required—a failure in the equipment and a failure in the process—to provide the necessary conditions for an explosion. Therefore, no limitation of energy in other than at normally operating contacts is required.

OTHER INTRINSIC SAFETY CODES

United Kingdom

British approval of intrinsically safe apparatus is given by the Ministry of Power for equipment to be used in mining and by the

Ministry of Labor for equipment to be used in other industries. Examination and testing, usually required, is performed by the Safety in Mines Research Establishment.

Although the British have been prolific in generating and publishing ignition data and have stated that an additional safety factor of 1.5 to 2 is normally used, no official definitions of fault considerations or specific constructional requirements have been published.

Criteria for ignition in resistive and inductive circuits are those developed using Break-Spark Apparatus No. 3 and the intermittent break apparatus, described in Chapter 4. The author knows of no public disclosure of criteria for capacitive circuits other than the Allsop-Guénault data referred to in Chapter 4.

Broad definitions and general requirements for intrinsically safe circuits and apparatus are given in British Standard 1259.

An intrinsically safe circuit is "a circuit in which any electrical sparking that may occur in normal working under the conditions specified by the Certifying Authority, and with the prescribed components, is incapable of causing ignition of the prescribed flammable gas or vapor."

Intrinsically safe apparatus is "apparatus that is so constructed that when installed and operated under the conditions specified by the Certifying Authority, any electrical sparking that may occur in normal working, either in the apparatus or in the circuit associated therewith, is incapable of causing an ignition of the prescribed flammable gas or vapor."

The term "intrinsically safe" as used in BS 1259 does not include ignition by means of glowing filaments of lamp bulbs, frictional sparking, or fusing of conductors.

The phrase "in normal working" is "intended to cover sparking that may, in normal use, be produced by breaking line current, or a short circuit across the lines, in the circuit that is required to be intrinsically safe. It is also intended to cover sparking that may be produced under any condition of fault which, in the opinion of the Certifying Authority, might arise in practice."

This approach to defining the conditions under which the circuit must be safe is similar to that taken in RP12.2 except that because a single testing agency is always used, the fault requirements are not specifically listed.

The author concludes, based on discussions with those who have dealt with the British Authorities in these matters, that in most cases a circuit or apparatus which is "intrinsically safe" per RP12.2 will also be "intrinsically safe" per BS 1259. It may not be true, however, that a British-approved system would be intrinsically safe per RP12.2 without ignition testing. Any differences in view regarding constructional requirements result from the fact that the British have a single responsible Testing Authority with continuity of history and responsibility. This authority is therefore able to rule safely that certain combinations of faults are not likely to occur under the normal conditions of operation of the equipment. RP12.2, on the other hand, prepared for general use, might negate a British-approved circuit because of the "no two fault" criterion. It should be emphasized that this difference in degree is still only of concern in those cases where circuits or equipment are being approved as intrinsically safe without test. The Safety Enforcement Authority may, at his own discretion, determine for himself the likelihood of any failure or combination of failures under the conditions of operation known to him.

Certification in the United Kingdom is based on examination and/or test by the Testing Authority, the Ministry of Power. Certificates will be issued by the Ministry of Power for mining applications or the Ministry of Labor for applications other than mining.

Table 9-1, based on Table 1 in BS 1259, shows the classifications of gases and vapors used for intrinsic safety certification. Note that the classifications are different from those used in British Standard 229 for the purposes of flameproof equipment. Approximately one-third of the gases and vapors listed were subjected to test. The remainder were classified on the basis of similarity of chemical properties and structure.

Testing of an apparatus or circuit for intrinsic safety is carried out using the representative gases listed below. All percentages are by volume.

Class 1	8.3% methane–air
Class 2c	3.9% pentane–air
Class 2d	7.8% ethylene–air
Class 2e	21% hydrogen–air
Class 2f	8.7% acetylene–air or other representative gas

Testing involves 200 operations under each test condition of Break-Spark Apparatus No. 3, or the intermittent break apparatus, or both. No ignitions shall occur with currents 50-100% in excess of the current in the normal operating condition. The higher margin will be required where it is reasonably practicable.

West Germany

The material which follows represents the author's understanding of the Sections of VDE 0170/0171d2:65 pertaining to intrinsic safety.

German practice is to require examination by the Physikalisch-Technische Bundesanstalt. The test apparatus to be used is that described in Chapter 4 as the PTB apparatus.

Certification will be either unrestrictedly intrinsically safe, tested with 21% hydrogen–air mixture, or restricted to a specifically named material.

The German approach appears to require energy to be limited to safe values after one fault, i.e., if components are added to restrict energy levels, there must be two, each of which is sufficient alone. Rectifiers and transistors may be loaded to no more than $\frac{2}{3}$ rated current and $\frac{2}{3}$ rated peak inverse voltage. Zener diodes may be operated at no more than $\frac{1}{2}$ rated current. Capacitors which determine intrinsic safety must be vacuum-tight, rated at 1500 V AC test voltage minimum, and be operated at less than $\frac{1}{3}$ rated voltage.

Exceptions to the requirement of two protective devices are components which are not likely to fail, such as wirewound resistors by shorting, and transformers of especially reliable design.

The minimum spacing in air, or creepage distance, between intrinsically safe and nonintrinsically safe circuits is 0.24 in. (6 mm). If connection between two portions of the intrinsically safe circuit would nullify safety, the same spacing requirement applies. The spacing may be reduced to 0.08 in. (2 mm) if the conductors are embedded in casting resin.

Terminal connections for equipment with both intrinsically safe and nonintrinsically safe circuits are to be made preferably in separate compartments. If located within the same compartment, they must be separated by at least two in. (50 mm) or separated by a suitably strong barrier.

Printed circuits must meet the minimum creepage distance requirement stated above except that the spacing between two conductors may be reduced to $\frac{1}{3}$ the stated value if a suitable protective layer is used.

Insulation between intrinsically safe circuits and ground must withstand a test of 500 V. Conductors in equipment containing both intrinsically safe and nonintrinsically safe wiring must withstand a 2000 V AC test in the nonintrinsically safe portion of the circuit, and an 800 V AC test in the intrinsically safe portion of the circuit.

Testing will be carried out using at least 1000 sparks of both polarities in DC circuits and 5000 sparks in AC circuits. Current or voltage levels during the test will be 50% greater than the highest obtainable with the equipment in normal working order but with external leads grounded, shorted, or opened; or that obtainable in the event of one fault, or one causally related train of faults. No ignition must occur. If failure of a voltage- or current-limiting resistor makes itself apparent, testing may be carried out without further increasing current.

Canada

CSA is considering an intrinsic safety regulation patterned after BS 1259, though it may differ in some details. It contemplates testing and examination by CSA Testing Laboratories and, at least at the present time, does not give specific, constructional require- ments for intrinsically safe apparatus and circuits.

United States Coast Guard

The USCG is proposing to adopt a safety regulation for marine service, particularly tankers, including the concept of intrinsic safety. Though it has not yet been officially adopted, it is likely to be similar to ISA RP 12.2.

Chapter 10

Evaluation of Systems for Intrinsic Safety

GENERAL CONSIDERATIONS

Evaluation of a system, i.e., equipment and associated wiring, to determine whether it is intrinsically safe in accordance with the requirements of ISA Recommended Practice RP12.2, is not, and cannot be, a "cookbook" procedure. ISA RP12.2 adequately states the essential energy limitations and specifies the considerations of failure against which to judge the system. However, it is not practical to list all possible specific constructional features which would render a particular mode of failure highly improbable or "for all practical purposes" impossible. The requirements of RP12.2 must be applied to a particular system with judgment. This judgment must be based on knowledge of the technology underlying the specific requirements of RP12.2. This is emphasized in RP12.2, paragraph 2.4:

"This Recommended Practice is intended to promote uniformity among specialists. It is intended that it be applied only by those who have carefully studied the subject. This Recommended Practice is not an instruction manual for untrained persons."

A similar assumption of responsible knowledgeability on the reader's part is recognized even in such a relatively detailed document as the National Electrical Code. In article 90-1(c) it states, "This Code is not intended as a design specification or an instruction manual for untrained persons."

Before attempting to evaluate a system for intrinsic safety one should ask himself, "Am I sufficiently familiar with the background of RP12.2 to make this analysis?" If this question cannot be answered in the affirmative, without reservations, it is strongly recommended that a qualified consultant be retained to make the analysis.

STEPS IN ANALYZING A SYSTEM

When analyzing a system to determine whether it is intrinsically safe it is convenient to divide the analysis into the following steps:

a. Determine which part of the system is to be classified intrinsically safe.
b. Evaluate energy levels in the portion of the system to be classified intrinsically safe, assuming that the entire system is in its normal operating condition.
c. Evaluate the energy levels in the portion of the system which is to be classified intrinsically safe under fault conditions without regard for constructional features of the device.
d. Where necessary, modify the conclusions of step (c) by consideration of the constructional features of the equipment.

This order of analysis assumes that either current and voltage levels in step (b) are found to be of sufficiently low value, or tentative corrective changes in circuitry are made before proceeding. If evaluation through steps (a), (b), and (c) shows the system to be intrinsically safe it is not necessary to consider constructional features. This not only saves considerable time in making the analysis, but also removes many judgment factors from the analysis. Also, only those constructional features which might alter the conclusions of step (c) need be considered. Analysis of other constructional features is unnecessary because the energy levels have been shown to be safe without concern for construction.

DETERMINING WHICH PART OF THE SYSTEM MUST BE INTRINSICALLY SAFE

Few systems have all equipment and wiring located in a Division 1 area, where the principle of intrinsic safety would be applied. Almost every electrical system receives power from equipment located in a nonhazardous or Division 2 location. At the very least a system will usually transmit signals to equipment located in other areas. Since it is not necessary and not economical (and very often impractical) to make equipment which is to be installed in a Division 2 or nonhazardous area intrinsically safe, only that portion of the system in the Division 1 area should be considered for intrinsic safety.

CIRCUIT ANALYSIS—NORMAL OPERATING CONDITIONS

Normal operation includes opening, shorting, or grounding of that connecting wiring between enclosures in the intrinsically safe portion of the system which is normally installed by the user and over which the equipment manufacturer has no direct control. If the system is intrinsically safe this wiring need not be in conduit or in MI cable. It may be lightly insulated wiring. This connecting wiring is therefore presumed to be susceptible to damage. Its terminal connections are assumed to be susceptible to shorting, opening, or grounding during the expected life of the installation.

The steps to be followed in analyzing the circuit under normal operating conditions are as follows:

a. Draw a complete system diagram, showing the value of all components in all of the equipment connected to that portion of the circuit which is intended to be intrinsically safe.

b. Indicate on the diagram the maximum values of circuit voltages and currents without considering shorts, opens, or grounds in the wiring, but assuming maximum supply voltage.

c. Compare the current through each inductor and the voltage across each capacitor with the values on the reference curves in RP12.2 (similar to those included in Chapter 9) applicable to the gas or vapor involved. Capacitors in parallel or inductors in series must be summed and treated as a single component. If the currents and voltages are less than 25% of those given in the reference curves, continue the analysis. If any current or voltage is greater than 25% of the value from the reference curves, the circuit cannot be regarded as being intrinsically safe without ignition testing. However, a tentative alteration of circuit constants or addition of a protective element should be considered. Circuit changes or constructional features to make the system intrinsically safe cannot be finalized until the analysis has considered both normal and fault conditions. Further consideration of this same portion of the circuit under fault conditions may show additional protection to be required. It is especially helpful when analyzing a system to record the steps in tabular manner. An example is given later in this chapter. Recording each step in the analysis gives greater assurance that important steps have not been omitted. The tabular presentation also makes it easier to use early calculations in later steps to save time.

d. Compute the worst case voltage at each capacitor and current through each inductor, considering shorting, grounding, or opening of external connecting wires, separately or in combination. Compare these values with those derived from the reference curves as in step (c). Should any values be above those which are derived from the reference curves, make a tentative selection of protective element or alter the circuit constants and continue circuit analysis under fault conditions.

CIRCUIT ANALYSIS—FAULT CONDITIONS

In analyzing a system under fault conditions it is necessary to consider all probable combinations of faults which can increase energy levels in the intrinsically safe portion of the system. It does not matter whether the fault occurs in the intrinsically safe or in a nonintrinsically safe portion of the system. An equipment fault in the Division 2 area which, for example, could connect the power line to wires entering a Division 1 area quite obviously would render a system unsafe.

Compute voltages and currents at capacitors and inductors for the worst case combination of two component or wiring failures, in addition to opening, shorting, or grounding of external wiring. No value shall exceed 50% of that read from the reference curves (25% if the circuit has a normally operating contact). This step in most cases represents the greatest part of the effort required in the analysis, since in most cases a large number of possible fault combinations must be evaluated before the worst case can be determined.

F. L. Maltby has suggested a very useful aid to reduce the amount of labor involved in considering the possible effects of a number of faults in one portion of the system, which the author has restated in general terms below.

Let a system be divided so that to one side of the dividing line lies equipment or circuitry A and to the other side lies equipment or circuitry B connected to equipment A by wires.

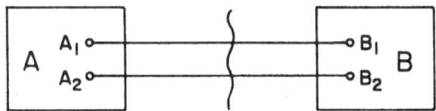

If: The number of connecting wires is two, connecting A_1 to B_1 and A_2 to B_2, and A contains only passive elements; I is the maximum current which can flow in the loop $B_1A_1A_2B_2$ when A_1 and A_2 are tied together and faults are presumed in B_1; V is the maximum voltage which can appear between B_1 and B_2 if the lines are open circuited;

And: Current I flowing through all inductances of equipment A in series is below the value derived from the reference curve; voltage V appearing across all capacitors in equipment A connected in parallel is below the value derived from the reference curve;

Then: Further consideration of individual fault combinations in A is not required.

For situations where equipment A is not passive, but contains sources, the above rule can be modified. The current I is taken as the sum of the short-circuit current of the source in A plus the current at A_1A_2 as defined above without regard for sign, and V is taken as the sum of the maximum open-circuit voltage of the source in A plus the maximum voltage at B_1-B_2 without regard for sign.

If A contains only passive elements but there are more than two wires connecting it to B, and if the currents in the connecting wires and the open-circuit voltages between all pairs of terminals at B are summed as above without regard for sign, the rule may be applied. However, for this and other complex cases it may be simpler to use some other rationale for showing that currents and voltages in A are maintained at safe levels. In a system with many interconnections, but where B contains a single source and A is passive, the system will be safe for any situation if the maximum open-circuit voltage of the B source and its short-circuit current are within limits after lumping all C's and L's respectively in A.

RE-EVALUATION OF THE SYSTEM TAKING INTO ACCOUNT CONSTRUCTIONAL FEATURES

Frequently steps (b) and (c) in the analysis of the system under normal and fault conditions will disclose that there are, at least on paper, one or more combinations of faults which will cause currents or voltages to exceed the specified limit values. In many cases it is possible that prudent construction of the equipment may render this required combination of failures so improbable that the combination need not be considered as a fault. ISA RP12.2 does not attempt to specify all ways in which prudent mechanical design will render a fault improbable. This approach would make RP12.2 a design specification of limited useful life and value. Principles for judging constructional features which will render a given fault highly improbable (so unlikely that it can be ignored) are summarized below:

a. The required combination of failures includes failure of a component in a manner inconceivable with regard to the component's construction and use. When this condition exists, the component is a "highly reliable component" as defined by RP12.2. The circuit will be intrinsically safe if no other single failure in combination with failure of this component will raise currents or voltages above the limit levels.

b. When the construction of the equipment is such that grounding of one portion of the circuit or connection of it to another point of the circuit is inconceivable, the fault can be considered not to be possible.

IMPORTANT CAUTION: Safety by construction is not to be indiscriminately applied. The fault must be of essentially zero probability in consideration of the following factors:

1. If the equipment is designated "intrinsically safe", maintenance operations and trouble-shooting procedures can be assumed to be carried out with little concern for explosion hazard.
2. Construction must be such that dropped tools, misapplied screwdrivers, test prods, etc., cannot significantly raise the probability that the fault will occur.

It is important to note that though constructional features must protect against accidental occurrences, even those of quite low probability, it is not required that they protect against deliberate circumvention.

Some common examples of constructional safeguards are summarized below.

Isolation of Line Voltage

In almost every intrinsically safe system it is necessary to protect against contact between power sources of relatively unlimited energy and connecting wires leading from a nonhazardous or Division 2 location into the intrinsically safe part of the system. This situation is shown schematically as follows:

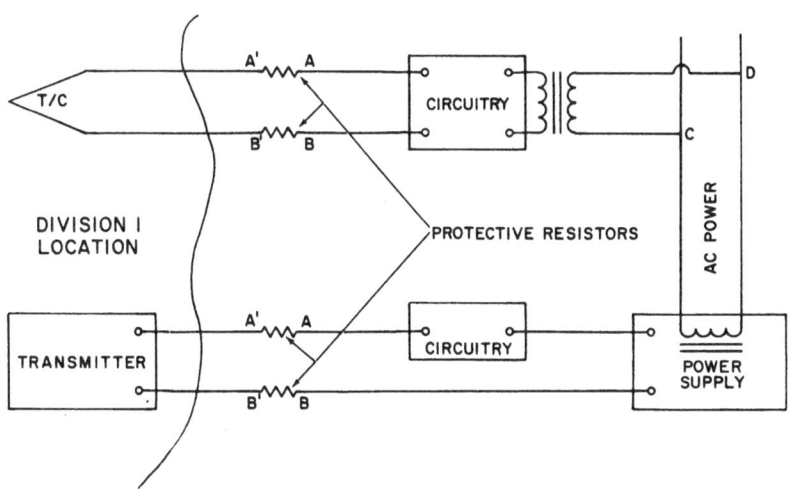

Frequently protective devices such as resistors can be installed in the location shown, so that energy in the part of the system in the Division 1 location cannot exceed permissible levels even if points

A and B are connected to points C and D. However, only the constructional features of the equipment located in the Division 2 area can assure that the probability that C and D will be connected to A' and B' is essentially zero. In many cases the circuitry is such that even without protective resistors no conceivable pair of faults could raise the energy level to the left of A' and B' above permitted values, if the construction prevents direct connection of A' and B' to C and D.

RP12.2 provides that insulated wires which are tied down so that they do not touch one another can be considered to have essentially zero probability of failure. For such wires to short, the insulation on each wire must fail and the tie-down means on one must fail—a total of three failures. A barrier may be substituted for the tie-down means. Some special considerations in protecting the intrinsically safe portion of wiring from connection to power lines or other high-energy level wiring are described below.

Internal Wiring

In internal wiring of a device, separation will usually be considered satisfactory if insulated conductors are firmly tied down so that they do not cross and if the high-energy-level wiring is not coupled in cables together with the intrinsically safe wiring. The spacing required is determined by ascertaining the necessary conditions in the particular design to ensure that the wires will not come together. Additional insulation or a barrier should be used in doubtful cases. Common cabling of power leads and intrinsically safe leads may sometimes be safe if the power leads are enclosed within a shield, so that the power leads can never raise the potential of the intrinsically safe leads. In most cases the shield must be grounded.

Terminal Blocks

Isolating by construction would normally be considered satisfactory if the power or other nonintrinsically safe connections are brought out on separate terminal boards at least two inches away from intrinsically safe terminal connections. A physical barrier is a more conservative, but not necessarily safer design. Construction of terminal blocks and the barrier must be such that, should external wiring come loose from the terminal screws, contact between the intrinsically safe wiring and the power wiring is highly improbable.

Transformer Construction

RP12.2 does not specify constructional features for transformers which couple an ignition-capable circuit to another circuit, a portion of which may be intrinsically safe. The construction requirements, however, must satisfy the fundamental principle that no two failures shall raise the current or voltage levels in the intrinsically safe portion of the circuit above the values determined from the reference curves. Frequently, in equipment connected to a power line, the power transformer is the only practical limiting component. The paragraphs which follow emphasize those features of transformer construction which are of importance in determining whether a transformer is a reliable isolating device. In the author's knowledge this material has not been codified anywhere, although VDE 0170/0171 contains specifications on bobbin construction.

Most commercial power transformers are of shell-type construction with "stick"-wound coil assemblies. A typical transformer is sketched in Figure 10-1. The coil assembly into which the core laminations are interleaved is usually wound simultaneously with many others. A cardboard insulating tube of rectangular cross section serves as a mandrel upon which the first layer of insulated wire is wound. As each layer of wire is completed it is additionally insulated by wrapping with insulating paper. Extra layers of paper may be added between windings. Copper shields sandwiched between insulating paper may also be wound between windings. When all windings are completed the start and finish ends of all windings are usually brought to the outside of the coil assembly, taped, and soldered to leads or to lugs. End bells may be added after stacking of the laminations in order to prevent mechanical damage to the windings.

The presence of an insulated and grounded shield very effectively prevents the two windings which it separates from being tied together by insulation failure. The exception is when both windings come into contact with the shield, but they are both then tied to ground, which is a safe situation. To raise the energy level on the secondary of a power transformer constructed in this fashion

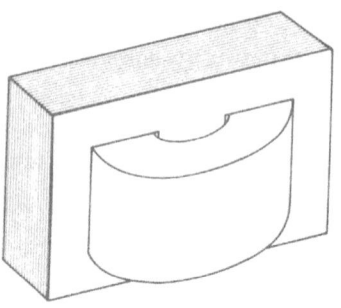

CROSS SECTION OF CORE

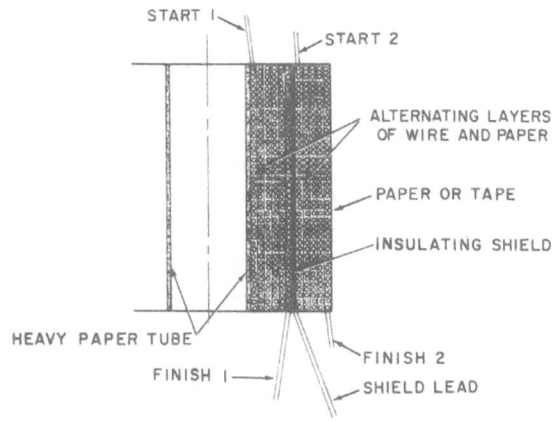

Fig. 10-1. Shell type transformer.

requires two insulation failures, one between each winding and the shield, plus a third failure, an open in the shield-ground connection. However, such a transformer constructed in the usual fashion is not safe. The primary and secondary winding ends are often run together to the outside of the coil assembly where leads may be attached and run through a single opening in the end bell. Isolation of primary and secondary leads is not guaranteed because insulation failure can allow primary and secondary leads to contact each other at the outside of the coil assembly.

For safety, in an intrinsically safe circuit the primary and secondary leads must be separated and secured in place. Extra insulation and/or encapsulation may be used. An economical way is to use fiber insulating tubes which are taped in the assembly at

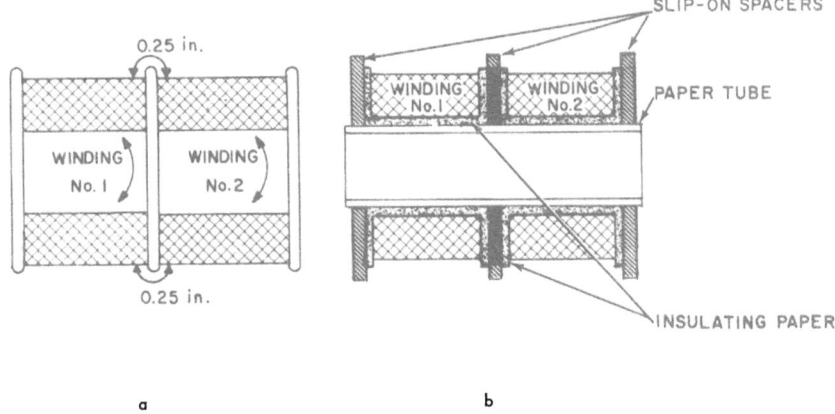

Fig. 10-2. Bobbin-wound coils. a) molded bobbin; b) fabricated bobbin.

the start and finish of a winding to provide extra protection for leads. The tubes also provide passage for bringing leads from the two windings to opposite ends of the assembly without being run adjacent to other leads or windings. The two sets of leads may be run through different holes in the end bells. Insulation failure on both sets may tie the two windings together through the end bells, but if the end bell and the core are grounded, such failure would be safe. These and other constructional techniques used in building very high voltage transformers, where corona and leakage between primary and secondary are problems, can be effectively and safely used in isolating transformers for intrinsically safe circuits.

Bobbin-wound coil assemblies in shell type transformers also can be constructed to offer safe isolation of primary and secondary windings. German specification VDE 0550, for example, recongnizes that two sorts of bobbin construction may be used, a molded bobbin or a built-up bobbin. If a molded bobbin such as is shown in Figure 10-2a is used, the fixed molded barrier between primary and secondary is presumed to be adequate as long as the creepage distance along the barrier from one winding to another is at least $^{1}/_{4}$ in. (6 mm). If the barrier is slid onto a mandrel or tube, then additional channel-shaped insulation must be used to guarantee isolation, as shown in Fig. 10-2b. A hi-pot test of 4000 V for 1 min. is required.

If either type of core construction is used, the windings and/or external circuitry must be constructed so that no pair of failures

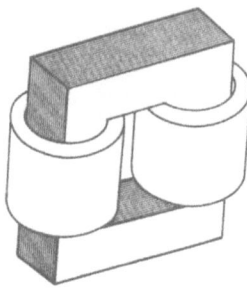

Fig. 10-3. Core type transformer.

will cause heating and degradation of the insulation to the extent that constructional safeguards are vitiated by catastrophic thermal failure.

Core type construction permits the use of commercial-grade "stick"-wound coil assemblies, and requires only that leads from the windings be well insulated and positively separated from one another. Such a transformer is sketched in Figure 10-3. If the core is grounded, insulation failures can connect the primary and secondary windings together only at ground potential, which is safe.

High-voltage (hi-pot) testing is conventionally used to determine whether windings are adequately isolated from one another and from shields, core, etc. Triple-voltage, triple-frequency testing, though less common, offers a valuable tool for checking the integrity of the windings as well as checking isolation between windings. The transformer is tested at no-load by applying 300%-rated primary voltage at 300%-rated frequency. Any leakage paths are subjected to 300% rated stress, but the flux density is close to design value, so that excessive currents do not flow. Weak spots in interlayer or interwinding insulation will cause abnormally high primary current to flow.

IMPORTANT CAUTION:

The foregoing discussion of transformer construction has dealt only with primary–secondary isolation. Such isolation trans- formers are not intrinsically safe transformers in the spirit of British Standard 1538 and must not be confused with them. Intrinsically safe transformers of the sort described in BS 1538 must, in addition to providing adequate isolation between primary and secondary windings, be constructed to limit the energy which can be transformed and to have especially low leakage inductance at power line frequency.

SEPARATION OF CIRCUITS IN GENERAL

The techniques discussed earlier for isolating line voltage from intrinsically safe circuits can be employed anywhere in the system to isolate one portion of the circuit from another. Some specific cautions are required in the following constructions:

a. Printed Circuit Board. Conductors on printed circuit boards which are coated with insulating varnish and which are protected from mechanical damage can usually be considered as being separated and securely tied down. However, connectors, terminals, and uninsulated leads of components mounted on the board normally represent the points of highest probability of accidental interconnection of circuitry. Component leads, terminals, and connectors must be so separated or insulated that it is inconceivable that a dropped tool or a misplaced piece of wire could cause a hazardous connection.

b. Connectors and Plugs. It is to be assumed that any leads entering the connector or plug are capable of being shorted to any other lead unless the connector construction makes the assumption ridiculous, as in some in-line printed circuit connectors. Assembly of most commercial connectors requires bare leads in very close proximity, or highly stressed insulation at the point where the bundle of leads enters the connector. Migration of wires within the insulation so that they eventually short is possible under these conditions. If individual leads are spaced and carefully insulated, particularly if leads are held in place with potting compound, the general rule may be excepted. The dangerous consequences of wire migration may be minimized by judicious use of grounded shields.

ISOLATION BY POTTING OR ENCAPSULATION

Many devices use large electrolytic capacitors which can be charged to voltages considerably in excess of those permitted by the reference curves. If one treats such a capacitor as an infinite source, i.e., a battery of the same voltage, the circuit can be made safe by ensuring that the capacitor always discharges through a limiting resistor. This resistor must limit the discharge current to the permissible level for zero inductance circuits of that supply voltage. This protection is effective only if the protective resistor cannot be shorted out, and the connection between the resistor and the capacitor cannot be shorted to another point in the circuit or grounded, permitting the capacitor to discharge through a path not including the protective resistor. An effective way of ensuring positive protection is to encapsulate the resistor and capacitor so that only one resistor and one capacitor lead are brought out of the potted assembly. Because the critical joint between the capacitor and resistor is safely embedded in the encapsulating material, there is no way that the joint can be shorted to another portion of the circuit. Such a failure can be considered impossible.

INDUCTANCE AND STORED ENERGY IN FERROMAGNETIC CORE INDUCTORS

Heretofore we have always referred to the stored energy in an inductance as being calculable from the expression

$$W = \tfrac{1}{2}LI^2$$

where W is stored energy in joules;
L is inductance in henries;
I is current in amperes.

This expression can only be used for calculating energy, however, in those cases where L does not change with current level. This condition is always satisfied in air-core inductors and is often approximately so in inductors with iron or other high-permeability cores. More often than not, the energy computed from known values of L for non-air-cored inductors bears little relationship to the amount of energy actually stored in the inductor. In short, the value of inductance measured by conventional methods has no necessary and predictable relationship to the energy stored in the inductor at a given current level. The stored energy at a specific current level can be measured or calculated only with great difficulty. If the geometry and constructional details of the inductor as well as the magnetic properties of the core are known, the amount of energy stored in the inductor can be estimated.

The problem of computing stored energy in a saturable core inductor can be best understood by recognizing that the expression $W = \tfrac{1}{2}LI^2$ is a special case of a more general expression, $W = V \int_0^B H\,dB$.

When μ, the permeability of the material, is constant and independent of H, then $B = \mu H$. This is the case in an air-core inductor. By definition the parameter L is equal to $N d\phi/dI$, the change of flux linkages in a magnetic circuit caused by changing the current which produces the flux.

Also,

$$d\phi = A\, dB$$

$$dI = \frac{l}{N}\, dH$$

where A is the area of the magnetic path;

l is the length of the magnetic path;

N is the number of turns through which the current I flows;

B is flux density;

H is magnetizing force;

$V = Al$ is the volume of the magnetic field, i.e., permeability of the magnetic material is assumed to be high with respect to air, so that all lines lie in the magnetic metal.

Therefore,

$$L = \frac{N d\phi}{dI} = \frac{AN^2}{l} \frac{dB}{dH}$$

For the air-core case where μ is constant,

$$L = \frac{AN^2}{l} \mu$$

$$W = V \int_0^B H\, dB = Al \int_0^H B\, dH = Al \int_0^H \mu H\, dH = \frac{Al}{2} \mu H^2$$

But

$$H = \frac{NI}{l}$$

So that

$$W = \frac{AN^2 \mu I^2}{2l} = \tfrac{1}{2} L I^2$$

When inductors have ferromagnetic cores, the permeability μ is not independent of H, and the differential form and the general integral must be used.

Since ϕ and B, and I and H are related by constants in any particular case it is convenient to continue the discussion on the basis of the familiar $B\text{-}H$ curve sketched below.

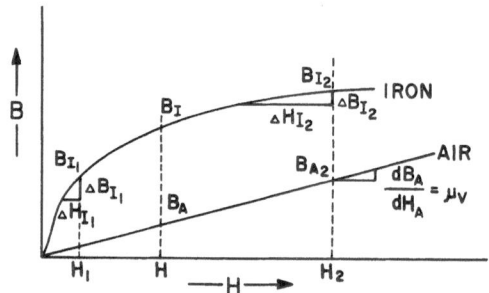

The straight line is a plot of the familiar relationship for air, $B = \mu_V H$, where μ_V is the permeability of free space. The curve marked "Iron" is drawn grossly out of scale, but is representative of core materials with nonlinear $B\text{-}H$ curves. At any magnetizing force H, the ratio B_I/B_A defines the relative permeability of the material, μ_r. For the material shown, since the $B\text{-}H$ curve becomes flat at high values of H the relative permeability decreases as H increases.

The slope of the $B\text{-}H$ curve at any point is the incremental permeability, $\Delta B_{I_2}/\Delta H_{I_2}$, $\Delta B_{I_1}/\Delta H_{I_1}$, or dB_A/dH_A. For air or other paramagnetic material the incremental permeability is constant. In ferromagnetic materials the incremental permeability may be low at low flux densities, increasing to as much as 800,000 Gausses per Oersted at higher flux densities and falling to very low values at saturation flux density.

As was noted above, the incremental permeability dB/dH is proportional to $Nd\phi/dI$, which is L, the inductance. With increasing values of H, ferromagnetic materials, as a class, display decreasing incremental permeability and, therefore, decreasing inductance. In modern square-loop materials the inductance may change by a factor of thousands, depending on the level of flux density.

The stored energy in the magnetic field, stated in integral form earlier in this section, is, for any value of H, proportional to the area under the $B\text{-}H$ curve. Quite obviously there is no simple relationship between L at $H = 0$ and the stored energy at $H = H_1$; nor is there any apparent relationship between L measured at $H = H_2$ and the stored energy for that value of H. Yet most AC bridges measure the inductance at $H_{avg} = 0$. Even special incremental inductance bridges, built for transformer and filter inductor measurements, which provide for measuring inductance at different levels of DC magnetization, offer no help. The low inductance measured if the inductor is operated on the flat portion of the B-H characteristic would give a very low estimate of the energy stored.

A certain, but often very conservative rationale is that if the inductance measured at $H_{avg} = 0$ is used as though it were the value of an air-core inductor, and the stored energy (or circuit current) is computed to be at a satisfactory level, there is no need for further concern.

Estimates of energy storage can be made using conventional magnetic circuit analysis if the e x a c t construction and material of the inductor are known. Small air gaps in inductors are frequently used to prevent DC currents from building up large values of H and causing low values of L. If air gaps are ignored in the analysis the estimated energy storage may be orders of magnitude too high.

Energy storage may be calculated using data from observed oscilloscope traces if the inductor is discharged through a resistor from a steady state current level. This method is tedious and approximate and is probably seldom worth the effort.

In any case in which the stored energy in a ferromagnetic core inductor is not obviously too small to be of consequence, ignition testing is strongly recommended. In general, ferromagnetic core inductors will be inefficient in releasing stored energy to the arc. Core losses dissipate energy and raise the circuit current required for ignition.

INDUCTANCE AND STORED ENERGY OF FERROMAGNETIC CORE TRANSFORMERS

Because the inductance of a transformer depends on the way in which it is connected in the circuit, transformers represent a slightly more complex problem than ferromagnetic core inductors. Much of what follows is applicable in principle to air-core transformers, but these are seldom of large enough size to present a safety problem. The transformer may be represented by the equivalent circuit sketched below.

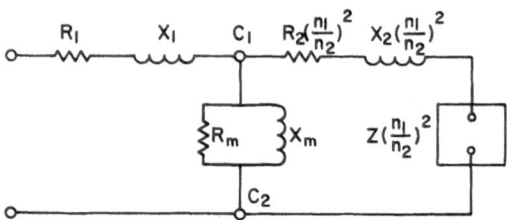

This equivalent circuit is the same as that found in any elementary text. Transformers with multiple secondaries can be represented by connecting the equivalent circuits of additional secondaries between C_1 and C_2.

Power transformers represent a particularly simple case. Usually the power transformer inductance is only of interest when viewed from the secondary winding. Unless the primary winding is connected to the power line, there is no hazard. When the primary winding is connected to the power line, the load Z in the equivalent circuit represents the source impedance of the power line. In any practical instrument system this impedance is usually so low that it can be presumed to be 0. For most transformers, if the load impedance is 0, the impedance looking into a winding is not much different from the sum of the series impedances,

$$R_1 + (n_1/n_2)^2 R_2 + j[X_1 + (n_1/n_2)^2 X_2]$$

The impedance represented by the center leg of the equivalent circuit is usually much higher than the winding impedances (it represents the magnetizing current and core losses, which are small compared to rated currents).

The inductance of a power transformer connected to the power line is therefore the leakage inductance of the transformer windings measured at low frequency and with appropriate direct currents flowing in the windings where applicable. Interpretation of the measurement is not subject to the same difficulties as in an iron-core inductor because the leakage inductance is caused mostly by flux lines in air. Therefore, the stored energy is more nearly proportional to inductance, as in an air-core inductor.

Coupling transformers, unless one winding is connected to a very low impedance source, pose the same problems as saturable core inductors, and are also subject to the influence of the reflected load impedance. The shunt impedance representing the magnetizing current can usually be ignored because it is high compared to all others in the circuit, including reflected load impedance. This is not always the case, however. It can certainly not be ignored if the load impedance, perhaps under fault conditions, can become very large or infinite as the result of an open circuit. In the open circuit case the transformer becomes an inductor, and all of the previously stated cautions apply.

In doubtful situations testing is highly recommended because losses in the transformer may make an apparently hazardous energy level quite safe. Of course, if no direct current flows in the windings and conventionally measured inductance values would be safe in an air-core inductor, the transformer would be safe.

PROTECTIVE ELEMENTS

Circuit elements which are depended upon to limit the level of current or voltage in a portion of a circuit may be series elements or shunt elements. Series elements limit current in a portion of the circuit. Shunt elements may divert current around a portion of the circuit to decrease the energy which can be released. Shunt elements may also be used to dissipate energy released by an inductor, which might otherwise be dissipated in an arc.

A significant and often crucial difference between series and shunt protective elements is that failure of series protective elements can always be arranged to be "fail-safe" so that any probable failure of the element is in the direction to reduce the current level. Shunt protective elements, on the other hand, can fail open-circuited and may therefore be unsafe. It is almost impossible to arrange shunt elements so that a pair of failures or, very often, just one failure cannot remove protection. Even more serious is the fact that shunt-element failure may be both unsafe and unrecognized. F. L. Maltby, in 1956, recommended that shunt elements not be employed to obtain safety, but only to increase it. The author feels that this philosophy is still generally applicable. In some circumstances redundant elements of conservative rating may be very carefully designed and built into a device, but complete loss of protection by these elements, whatever their number, should not, in his view, raise energy levels above the limiting values. In most situations the requirement of RP12.2 that no two faults shall raise the current or voltage levels above 50% of the value determined from the reference curves will prevent effective use of shunt elements except to increase safety under normal conditions. In British practice some shunt elements are recognized as effective limiting devices. However, the requirements of such devices are not documented, except for metal rectifiers, which are covered by British Standard 2031. The author does not know specifically to what extent and with what restrictions such devices are approved.

Series Protective Elements

Series resistors will be commonly used as protective elements in DC and AC circuits to limit the amount of current that can flow in the intrinsically safe portion of a circuit. Wirewound, single-layer elements on robust nonconducting mandrels and insulated with ceramic or other electrically and physically strong insulation can be mounted so that failure by shorting is too remote to be considered as a potential fault. Such resistors are sufficiently inexpensive that two can be used in series. Metal film construction also can be used to meet the requirement that failure by decrease in resistance be of essentially zero probability. Ordinary composition resistors must not be used. They can fail by decreasing in resistance.

It is likely that German regulations will stipulate that current-limiting resistors of 0.008 in. minimum wire diameter, embedded with windings secured against unwinding if a break occurs, may be used at half rated power.

Series capacitors are most likely to be used in devices such as liquid-level probes which operate at high frequency but low AC power level. A pair of capacitors in series can effectively isolate the probe circuit from DC voltages and currents of potentially incendive levels used in the measuring equipment located in a Division 2 or nonhazardous location. Capacitors such as silvered mica units or silvered ceramic units with leads brought out at opposite sides can be constructed and mounted to have zero probability of shorting. Even paper or plastic dielectric might be used, depending on the construction of the particular component. German requirements will likely be that the capacitor be operated at less than one-third rated voltage, that it withstand 1500 V test voltage, and be hermetically sealed.

Fuses and circuit breakers shall not be used to limit current. The time scale of ignition is in the $0-500\,\mu$ sec range, faster than these devices operate. The author knows of no tests indicating successful use of a fuse as a limiting element where a fixed resistor of the same resistance as the fuse would not also have been adequate. This is not to say that there are no exceptions, but until contrary test results are available, it must be assumed that fuses and circuit breakers are not effective energy-limiting devices.

Shunt Protective Elements

Shunt resistors, linear or nonlinear, may be effectively used to help dissipate the energy stored in an inductor. Though the data reported in Chapter 4 indicate the order of hazard reduction, in any circuit using shunt resistors for hazard reduction the amount of protection achieved must be determined by test. There are no analytical methods for estimating with accuracy the added safety contributed by a shunt element in terms of the inductance, the resistance of the shunted inductor, and the other circuit constants.

The construction of protective shunt resistors and the manner in which they are wired into a circuit is of great importance. The resistor must be of high quality, wound of heavy wire, with firmly anchored leads so that an open circuit is of essentially zero probability. When a resistor or other shunt element is used, the inductor itself must be of highly reliable construction so that an inductor lead cannot fail open and then ground or short to another part of the circuit. This could cause arcing without protection from the shunt element.

Shunt capacitors must meet the same general requirements as shunt resistors, in that construction must ensure that open circuits are of very low probability. As in the case of shunt resistors, the effectiveness of a particular arrangement has to be demonstrated by test because no analytical techniques are available. Evaluation of protective capacitors must include consideration of the fact that shunt capacitors will in some instances increase hazard, particularly those of moderate size (less than $1\,\mu$F), if slow or intermittent breaks occur.

Shunt rectifiers used to limit voltage developed by inductors in opening circuits and to dissipate their stored energy are installed in parallel with the inductor, so that current normally does not flow in the diode. If a break occurs in the circuit the voltage generated by the collapsing magnetic field in the inductor is conducted by the rectifier. Possible failure by open circuit is again the most important consideration in selecting a shunt rectifier. Modern germanium and silicon diodes have much lower forward voltage drop and much higher reverse leakage resistance than metal rectifiers of the type for which test data were reported in Chapter 4. Some have expressed concern that hole storage in some such rectifiers may delay transition from the nonconducting to the conducting state long enough to decrease their ability to prevent ignition. There are, however, very fast acting diodes available and it is doubtful that hole storage is a serious problem, if it is a problem at all. The efficacy of a particular diode must be shown by test. Any diode used must of course have adequate ratings for the expected environment, more than ample reverse voltage rating and forward current rating, and very reliable construction.

Series–Shunt Limiting Devices

Several combinations of series and shunt devices have been proposed for limiting current or voltage in a portion of a circuit. All have in common a series element to limit current, and a nonlinear element to limit voltage. Three varieties are sketched below. The connections to the safe circuit are to the right.

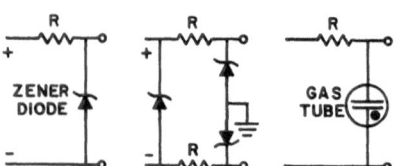

In most circuits today a Zener diode will usually be used as the voltage-limiting element. The Zener diode has a very high impedance until a critical voltage is reached, at which voltage the impedance is low and current is high. If two Zener diodes are connected back-to-back and the common connection is grounded, any voltage appearing between the two circuit conductors and ground will be limited in value. Zener diodes may also be used to limit voltage in AC circuits by connecting a pair of diodes rated above the peak value of normal working voltage back-to-back.

Copper Sleeves, Slugs, and Shorted Windings

In DC relays, DC force coils, or other inductive devices much of the energy stored in the inductance can be dissipated by a shorted turn in the coil structure. When such construction is used the aim is to provide a closed low-resistance path so that a collapsing magnetic field will induce current in the shorted turn. Not only is the stored energy dissipated in I^2R heat loss; but also, current flow in the shorted turn sets up a magnetic field in the same direction as that which caused initial current to flow, delaying the collapse of the field. In electromechanical devices slugs or rings of copper may provide such shorted turns. They need not be geometric turns; slugs or plates will allow eddy currents to flow to accomplish the same end. In wound coils a bare winding may be laid down and soldered together. The efficacy of any construction must be established experimentally.

ILLUSTRATIVE EXAMPLE: ANALYSIS OF A SYSTEM FOR INTRINSIC SAFETY

The example which follows illustrates analysis of a system for intrinsic safety. The system has in it many of the elements of a real measuring and control system. The system is not a real system, however, and represents no particular design.

The analysis is being made with respect to gases and vapors in the "Pentane" group. The analysis follows the steps previously presented. Typical simplifications and approximations which reduce the amount of work in the analysis are included.

Determination of the part of the system to be approved as intrinsically safe in this case poses no problem. The transmitter and transmission lines located in the Division 1 area must be intrinsically safe. The power supply and receiver located in the Division 2 location need only be suitable for that location. The effect of power supply and receiver failures on energy levels in the intrinsically safe portion of the system must, of course, be considered.

CIRCUIT ANALYSIS—NORMAL OPERATING CONDITIONS

The circuit illustrated in Fig. 10-4 shows the voltages applied to the circuit under nominal conditions. For intrinsic safety

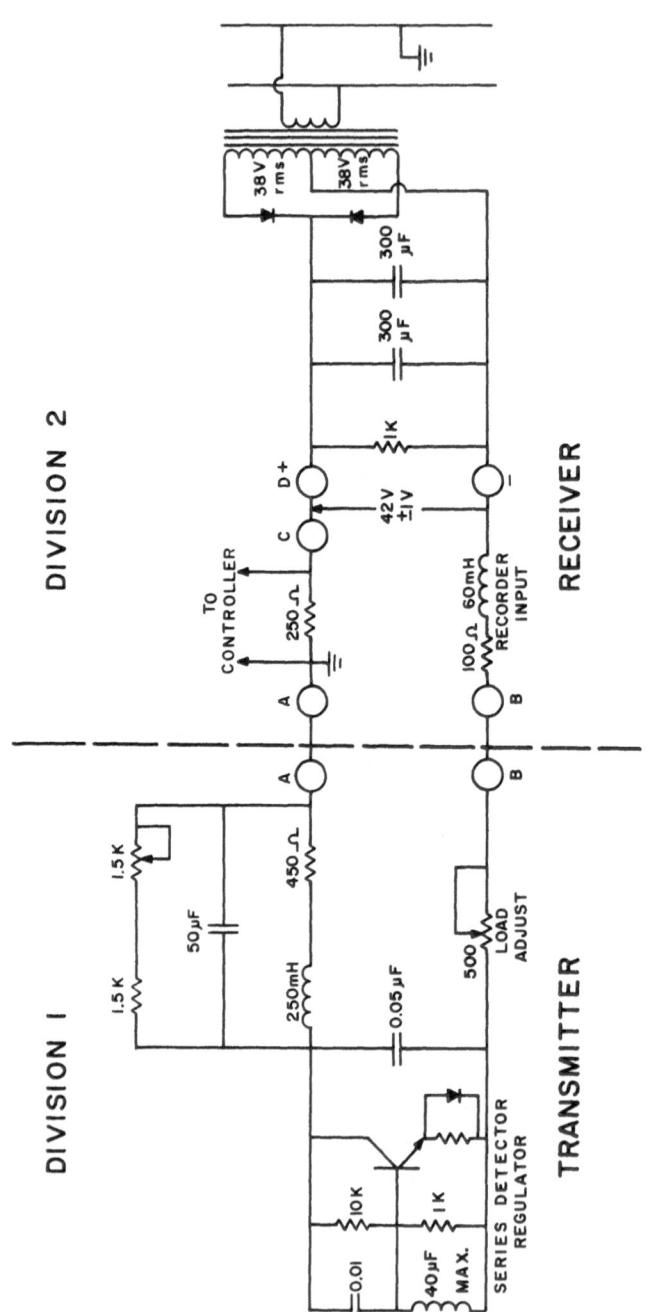

Fig. 10-4. System as analysis starts.

analysis the voltages used must be the maximum to be expected within the ratings of the system. In normal operation the regulated power supply voltage is assumed to reach 43 V if the line voltage goes to 120 V + 15%.

We will now evaluate circuit currents and voltages without taking into account that opens, shorts, and grounds are included in normal operation.

Because the load adjust pot, 500 Ω, is provided for field adjustment, in this analysis it is assumed that it is set at zero ohms. Except by replacing it with a fixed resistor, there is no way to guarantee that it will always be set at some predetermined value. To be conservative, therefore, we assume that its resistance is negligible.

An electromechanical transmitter of the type whose circuit is sketched above can draw current appreciably above its nominal current range during a transient, or if the input is overranged, but the current can certainly never exceed that determined by the supply voltage and series resistances alone.

The detector–regulator circuit will pass negligible current unless the voltage drop across it is at least 8 V, enough to turn on the transistor. In the calculations the drop across this element will always be assumed to be 8 V. In order to keep the example to reasonable length, it is assumed also that controller and recorder construction is such that there is no possibility of coupling energy into the transmitter circuit. In a real system, recorder and controller circuits must, of course, be considered carefully to determine their effect on current and voltage levels in the intrinsically safe circuit.

Table 10-1 details the steps taken to analyze the circuit under normal conditions. The procedure followed is to calculate circuit current or voltage under stated conditions, compare it with permissible values determined from the curves with applicable additional factor of safety from RP12.2, modify the circuit if necessary, and recalculate previous steps if the circuit modification requires it.

The effect of the two 3K pots shunting the 250 mH, 450 Ω coil is neglected in calculating current in order to simplify calculations. Any effect of the shunt resistors and capacitor on ignition capability of the inductor must be neglected in a paper analysis because it is not predictable.

TABLE 10-1. Circuit Analysis Under Normal Conditions

Step No.	Capacitor or inductance	Circuit condition	Calculated voltage or current	Permitted voltage or current	Conclusion
1	250 mH and 60 mH	Normal.	43.8 mA	23.7	Add 675 Ω between point A and 250 Ω controller input. Anticipating failure conditions, make this two 350 Ω resistors in series.
2	60 mH	Normal, Short A to B.	41 mA	62.5 mA	OK
3	60 mH	Normal, Ground B.	123 mA	62.5 mA	Move one 350 Ω resistor to other line between recorder input and point B.
4	60 mH	Normal, Ground B. Resistor moved.	61.4 mA	62.5 mA	OK

5	250 mH and 60 mH	Normal, Ground A.	30.5 mA	23.7 mA	Must add 325 Ω or reposition the fixed resistors. Reviewing steps 1-5 suggests that putting two 350 Ω resistors added in step 1 between C and D would be better. Recheck 1-5 for this condition.
1A	250 mH and 60 mH	Normal and two 350 Ω resistors,	23.4 mA	23.7 mA	OK
2A	60 mH	Normal. Short A to B, two 350 Ω resistors added.	41 mA	62.5 mA	OK
3A	60 mH	Normal and 2 resistors. Ground B.	41 mA	62.5 mA	OK
5A	250 mH and 60 mH	Normal. Ground A.	12.4 mA	23.7 mA	OK
6	50 μF	Normal. Short A to B.	10.5 V	4.75 V	Add series R, 2.8 Ω, to limit current as though capacitor were an infinite source.

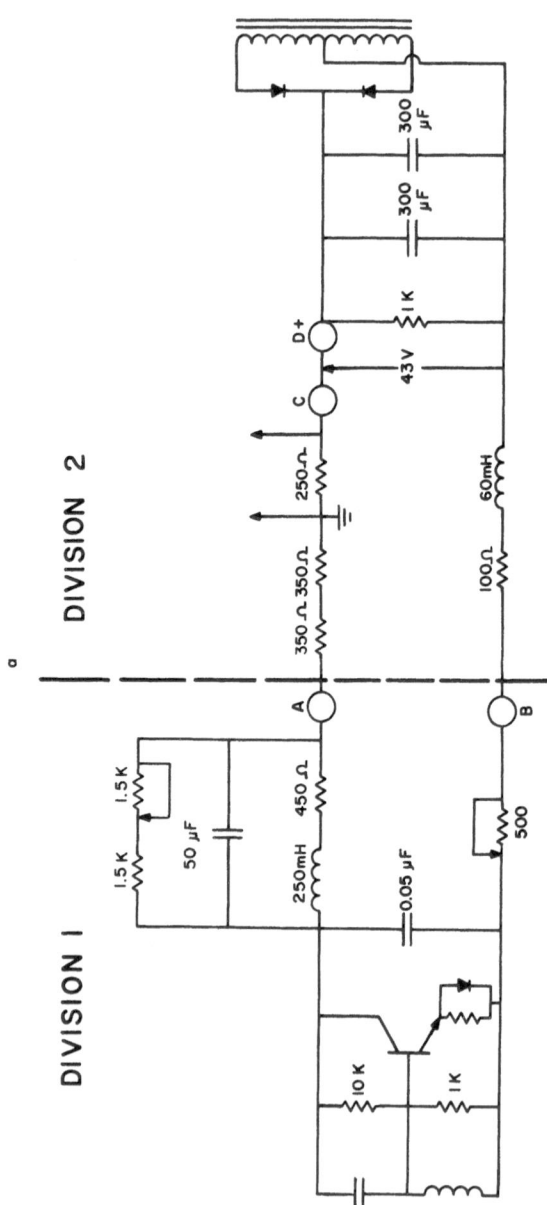

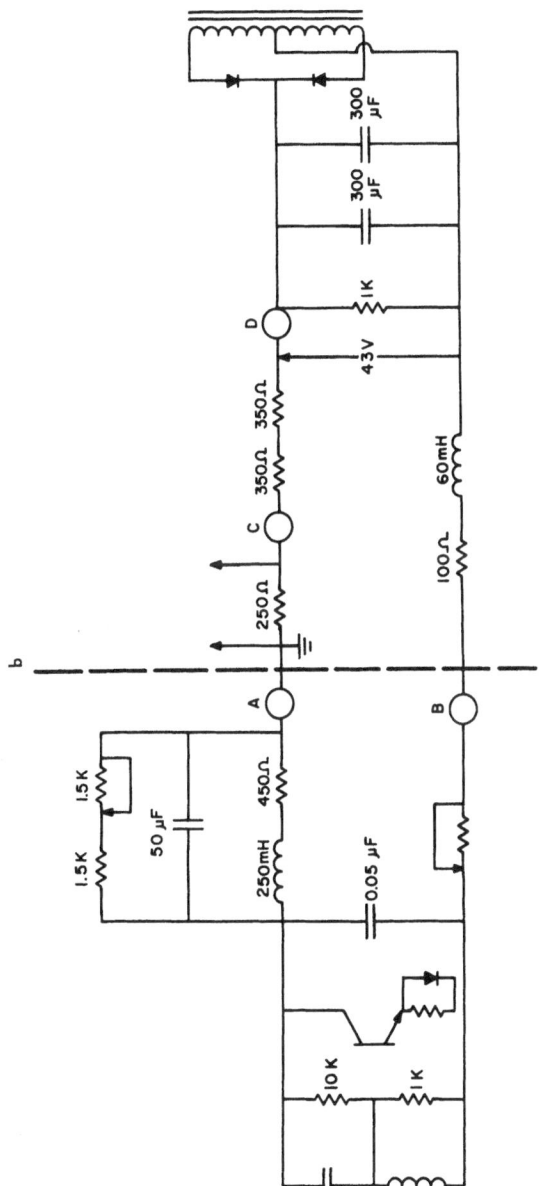

Fig. 10-5. a) System after step 1, Table 10-1; b) system after step 5, Table 10-1.

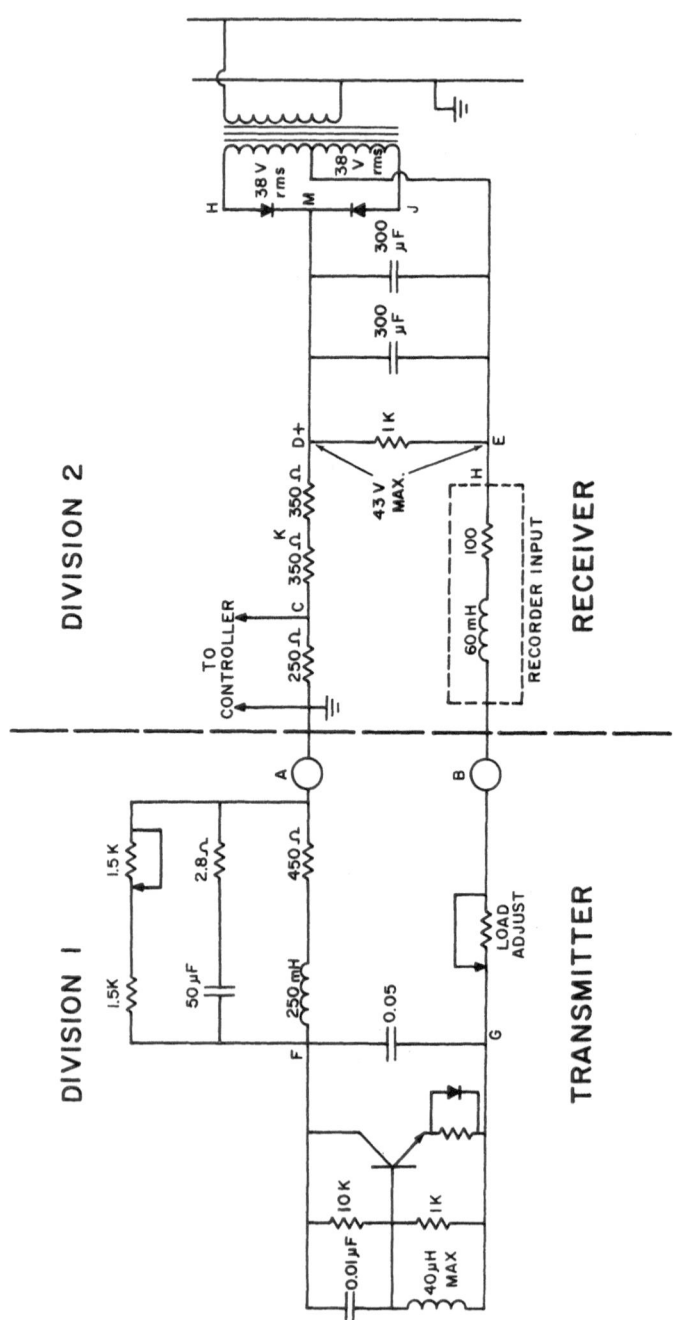

Fig. 10-6. System as analysis under fault conditions starts.

The calculations supporting Table 10-1 are given in Appendix 10-1.

CIRCUIT ANALYSIS—FAULT CONDITIONS

Even in the simple circuit being studied, consideration of all possible faults is time-consuming and wasteful of effort. The analysis continued below therefore uses conservative approximations as frequently as possible. These approximations are, however, always on the safe side.

We now redraw the circuit with added components suggested by the analysis under normal conditions, as in Table 10-1 (see Figure 10-6). The quickest way to show safety under fault conditions is to determine that, even if the transformer suffers a primary–secondary short, the system is safe if one additional fault occurred. Attention to wire routing and insulation would then be all that is required. Can this be done? At line voltage of 120 + 15%, peak voltage is 195 V.

Step 1 in Table 10-2 shows that a primary–secondary short in the transformer is not a safe condition, even without a second fault, unless series resistance in the circuit is increased greatly, or a shunt voltage-limiting element is added to the circuit at point D-E. Adding sufficient series resistance to limit current when a primary–secondary short occurs would defeat the normal function of the circuit. Between addition of a shunt limiting element and construction of the transformer so that it will not short, the author would choose the latter alternative because it is more reliable. For the remainder of the analysis, it will be assumed that the transformer will not suffer a primary–secondary short.

The highest possible voltage that can exist in the circuit if a primary–secondary short cannot occur is 78 V rms, but examination of the circuit shows that no pair of failures will cause this, which would be likely in a real device. For further analysis, we must therefore consider only the case where the voltage at D-E is 38 V rms or 53.7 V peak. We will assume that one failure (a filter capacitor open, for example) is required to cause the voltage to rise to this value, and will assess the safety of the circuit for the case of one additional failure.

Steps 2–5 in Table 10-2 show that any one additional failure beyond that assumed to be necessary to raise the voltage to 53.7 V

TABLE 10-2. Analysis Under Abnormal Conditions

Step	Capacitor or inductance	Condition	Calculated voltage or current	Permitted voltage or current	Conclusion
1	60 mH	Pri—sec Transformer short. Ground B.	186 mA	125 mA	Make pri—sec short essentially zero probability by proper construction of transformer.
2	60 mH and 250 mH	53.7 V at D-E. Ground D.	97.6 mA	47.4 mA	Move two 350 Ω resistors to line between recorder input and point E.
3	60 mH and 250 mH	53.7 V at D. Ground D. 350 Ω resistors moved.	43 mA	47.4 mA	OK
4	60 mH and 250 mH	53.7 V at D. Short H to J.	39.8 mA	47.4 mA	OK, but must fix construction so both 350 Ω resistors cannot be shorted. Make one 350 Ω highly reliable construction, and mount so can't be shorted.

5	60 mH	53.7 Ma at D. Ground B. Short H to J.	76.6 mA	125 mA	OK. This is worst case. Any other short can only short out 250 Ω controller input or bypass 60 mH coil.
6	60 mH	43 V at D. Ground B. Ground C. Short H to J.	95.5 mA	125 mA	OK. This is worst case because remaining 350 Ω is highly reliable and cannot be shorted out.
7	60 mH and 250 mH	43 V at D. Ground D. Short H to J.	38.9 mA	47.4 mA	OK
8	250 mH	Ground D. Short B to J.	43.7 mA	55 mA	OK
9	250 mH	Short B to J. Short F to G.	37.3 mA	55 mA	OK
10	0.05 μF capacitor	Any possible condition.	43 V	150 V	OK
11	50 μF capacitor	Open 250 mH coil. Short B to J.	35.8 max	9.5	Increase 2.8 Ω to 15 Ω.

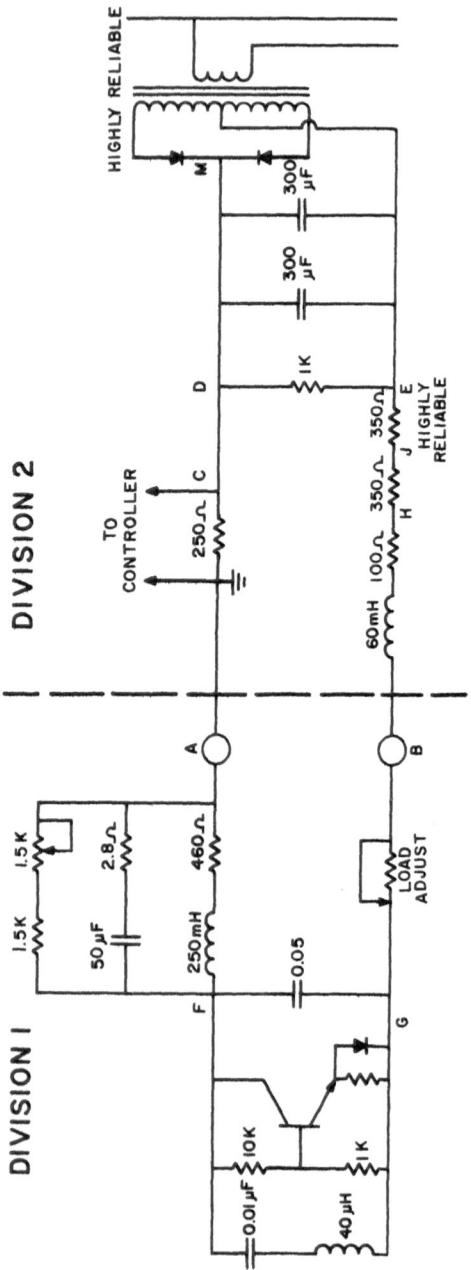

Fig. 10-7. Circuit after step 2, Table 10-2.

does not raise current levels above those permitted if the two 350 Ω resistors are relocated in the circuit and one is made highly reliable.

It is now necessary to assess the circuit for the case where the voltage at D-E remains normal at 43 V maximum, and two additional failures occur in the circuit.

Steps 6–9 in Table 10-2 show the analysis with respect to fault currents. No rearrangement or addition of resistors is required to make the circuit safe.

The one last check which must be made is the possible hazard of the 50 μF and 0.05 μF capacitors. The maximum voltage which can appear across the capacitor is when the 250 mH coil opens and B-J is shorted. Steps 10 and 11 show that the 0.05 μF capacitor presents no hazard, but the resistance in series with the 50 μF capacitor must be increased to 15 Ω to limit current should the capacitor be grounded.

The system, with all protective resistors properly located, is now as shown in Fig. 10-8.

Energy storage in the small capacitor and inductor in the transistor circuit was not considered because it is obviously so small compared to others considered that it adds no significant hazard.

Note that the foregoing analysis has not included consideration of other circuitry connected to the 100 Ω 60 mH receiver coil or the 250 Ω controller input resistor. It is implicit in this analysis, but would have to be explicit in an analysis of a real system, that construction effectively isolates these elements from sources of energy of magnitude great enough to be of concern in the part of the system studied. The analysis has also ignored such single failures as a short from F to J, which in a real system would require grounding of F, grounding of J, and opening of the controller ground. Additional fault conditions which could be evaluated by inspection were not included in Table 10-2 in order to keep the illustration to reasonable length and render it more representative of a real analysis.

DETERMINATION THAT A SYSTEM IS NONINCENDIVE

The determination as to whether a system is nonincendive is much simpler than determination as to whether a system is intrin-

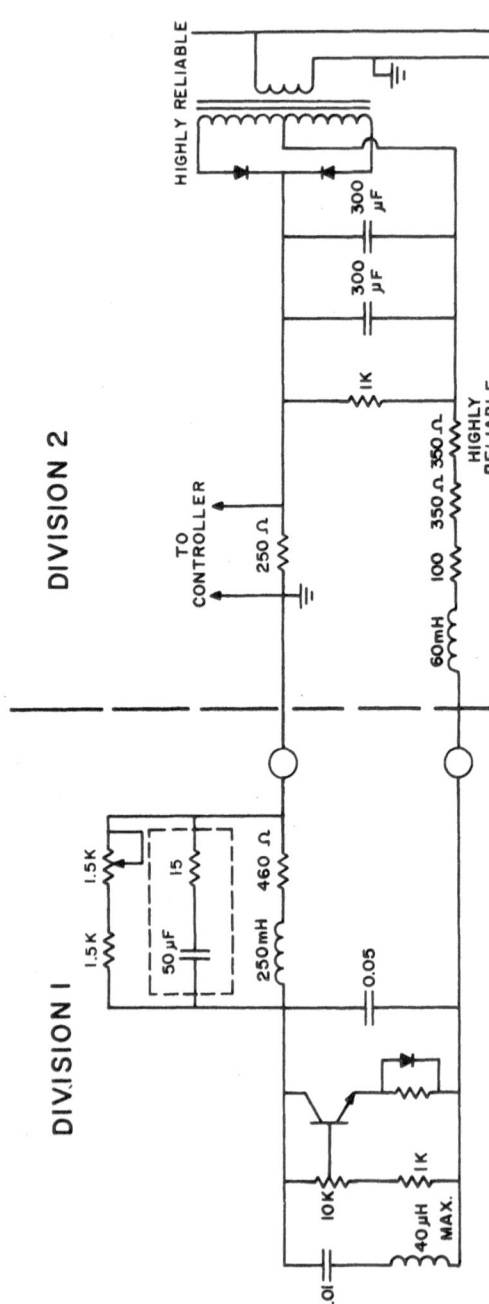

Fig. 10–8. System after analysis is completed.

sically safe. Only the currents and voltages in circuits which make and break under normal operating conditions must be considered; fault conditions need not be considered. Shorting, grounding, or opening of connecting wiring, which is considered a normal condition in intrinsically safe systems, need not be considered in non-incendive systems. Most industrial instruments may have only one or two circuits with normally operating contacts. Only the currents and voltages in these circuits must be compared to the reference curves with an additional factor of safety of 4. If the contacts are protected by oil immersion, sealing, or another method suitable for Division 2, the circuit need not be considered.

Plugs, switches, and adjustments used only during maintenance or calibration are not considered as arcing contacts. These would usually include disconnect plugs in cables, and span and zero adjustments. Power switches, Proportioning Band, Rate, and Reset settings, and Set Point adjustments would in most devices be considered normally operating controls, and, if not otherwise protected, must be evaluated as arcing contacts.

APPENDIX 10-1: CALCULATIONS FOR TABLE 10-1

Step 1. $$I = \frac{43 - 8}{250 + 450 + 100} = \frac{35}{800} = 43.8 \text{ mA}$$

From Fig. 9-1: Ignition current for 310 mH = 95 mA
Permitted current = 95 · 0.25 = 23.7 mA
Need total resistance = 35/0.0237 = 1475 Ω. Add 675Ω to circuit.

Step 2. $$I = \frac{43}{250 + 700 + 100} = \frac{43}{1050} = 41 \text{ mA}$$

0.25 × current from Fig. 9.1 = 0.25 · 250 = 62.5 mA.

Step 3. $$I = \frac{43}{250 + 100} = 123 \text{ mA}$$

Step 4. $$I = \frac{43}{250 + 100 + 350} = 61.4 \text{ mA}$$

Step 5. $$I = \frac{43 - 8}{250 + 450 + 350 + 100} = \frac{35}{1150} = 30.5 \text{ mA}$$

Permitted current is 23.7 mA, so must add 325 Ω in circuit.

Step 1A. $I = \dfrac{43 - 8}{250 + 450 + 700 + 100} = \dfrac{35}{1500} = 23.4$ mA

Step 2A. $I = \dfrac{43}{700 + 100 + 250} = \dfrac{43}{1050} = 41$ mA

Step 5A. $I = \dfrac{43 - 35}{700 + 100 + 450 + 250} = 23.4$ mA

Step 6. Max. voltage on capacitor $= \dfrac{(43 - 8)\,450}{100 + 250 + 450 + 700} = \dfrac{35 \cdot 450}{1500} = 10.5$ V

$0.25 \times$ voltage from Fig. 9.4 $= 0.25 \cdot 19 = 4.75$ V.

From Fig. 9.1 can have 10 A in resistive circuit at 24 V. With safety factor can have 2.5 A. Add 2.8 Ω in series with capacitor. Note that 8 V drop across detector–regulator makes this resistance a very conservative value, but in anticipation of failure conditions, this drop will be ignored.

APPENDIX 10-2: CALCULATIONS FOR TABLE 10-2

Step 1. $I = \dfrac{195}{350 + 350 + 250 + 100} = 0.186$ A

Step 2. $I = \dfrac{53.7}{450 + 100} = 0.0976$

(Approximate calculation, neglecting F-G drop and shunting of 250 mH coil.)

Step 3. $I = \dfrac{53.7}{450 + 100 + 700} = 0.043$

(This neglects drop across F-G, so is conservative.)

Step 4. $I = \dfrac{53.7 - 8}{450 + 100 + 350 + 250} = \dfrac{45.7}{1150} = 0.0398$

Step 5. $I = \dfrac{53.7}{350 + 100 + 250} = \dfrac{53.7}{700} = 0.0766$

Step 6. $I = \dfrac{43}{100 + 350} = \dfrac{43}{450} = 0.0955$

Step 7. $I = \dfrac{43 - 8}{100 + 450 + 350} = \dfrac{35}{900} = 0.0389$

Step 8. $\qquad I = \dfrac{43 - 8}{350 + 450} = \dfrac{35}{800} = 0.0437$

Step 9. $\qquad I = \dfrac{43}{250 + 450 + 350} = \dfrac{43}{1150} = 0.0373$

Step 10.

From Fig. 9–4, voltage is greater than 300 V. Permissible voltage greater than 150 V.

Step 11.

Capacitor Voltage = 43 · 3000/(250 + 3000 + 350) = 35.8 V maximum, neglecting 8 V regulator–detector drop.
From Fig. 9-4 permitted voltage is 19/2 = 9.5 V.
From Fig. 9-1 permitted current is 5/2 = 2.5 A at 42.5 V.
Increase series resistor to 15 Ω.

REFERENCES

1. Proceedings of 1960 Symposium on Safety for Electrical Istrumentation in Hazardous Areas, Instrument Society of America, Pittsburgh.
   Maltby, F. L., "History of ISA Committee on Hazardous Area Instrumentation."
   Hickes, W. F., "Intrinsic Safety."
2. "A Review of Electrical Research and Testing with Regard to Flameproof Enclosure and Intrinsic Safety of Electrical Apparatus and Circuits," Ministry of Fuel and Power, 1943, London.
3. National Electrical Code, Article 500.
4. British Standard 2031, "Metal Rectifiers for Intrinsically Safe Signaling and Control Circuits."
5. British Standard 1259:1958, "Intrinsically Safe Electrical Apparatus and Circuits."
6. British Standard 1975:1953, "Primary Cells and Batteries for Intrinsically Safe Bell Signaling Circuits in Coal Mines."
7. British Standard 1538:1949, "Intrinsically-Safe Transformers for Bell-Signaling Circuits."
8. British Standard Code of Practice CP 1003:1948, "Installation and Maintenance of Flameproof and Intrinsically-Safe Electrical Equipment."
9. Ministry of Fuel and Power Testing Memorandum No. 10, "Test and Certification of Intrinsically Safe Electrical Apparatus and Circuits."
10. IEE Conference Report Series No. 3, "Flameproofing, Intrinsic Safety, and Other Safeguards in Electrical Instrument Practice," April 27, 1962.
    Berz, I., "Protective Devices for Intrinsically Safe AC Circuits."
    Haig, Lister, and Gordon, "The Testing of Flameproof and Intrinsically Safe Electrical Apparatus."
    Redding, R. J., "Intrinsic Safety Practice in Industrial Instrumentation."
    Thomas, V. M., "The Design of Intrinsically Safe Apparatus for Use in Coal Mines: A Review of Data and Technique."
    Wells, G. M., "Intrinsically Safe Instrumentation in Coal Mining."
    Simons, Kögeler, and Bijl, "Safety of Electrical Instruments in the Oil Industry."

Chapter 11

Dust Hazards

NATURE OF THE DUST HAZARD

The development of an explosion in a dust cloud is not, in principle, different from the development of an explosion in a gas or vapor. The important concepts presented in Chapter 3 are therefore generally, though not specifically, applicable to both types of explosion.

Like gas or vapor mixtures, dust suspensions have a minimum ignition energy and a lower explosive limit. Pressures developed in dust explosions are of the same order as those in gas or vapor explosions.

The salient differences between dust explosions and gas or vapor explosions are attributable to the physical differences between the two systems. A dust cloud is a nonhomogeneous suspension of solid particles in a suspending medium, usually air. Ignition characteristics and the characteristics of a dust explosion depend on the chemical composition of the dust, the shape, size, and concentration of the dust particles, and the chemical composition of the suspending medium.

In the following paragraphs the author has attempted only to briefly summarize and illustrate the most important features of dust hazards. He strongly recommends that the reader who is seriously concerned with dust hazards should consult the reference documents. The Bureau of Mines literature, in particular, contains a wealth of data too voluminous to reproduce in a work of this sort. These documents are a ready reference library of information on dusts. To the author's knowledge, there is nothing comparable in the gas–vapor explosion literature.

INFLUENCE OF CHEMICAL COMPOSITION OF THE DUST

Chemical composition is of prime importance in determining minimum ignition energy, minimum explosive concentration, pressure developed by the explosion, rate of pressure rise, and ignition temperature. However, though the range of values of these characteristics within a class of dusts covers several orders of magnitude, there are not substantial differences between classes. Whether one is considering metallic dusts, carbonaceous dusts, plastic or chemical dusts, or agricultural dusts, the following values are typical:

Minimum ignition energy . . . . . . .5 mJ and higher
Minimum explosive concentration .0.02 oz/ft^3 and higher
Maximum pressure developed. . . .30−130 psi
Rate of pressure rise . . . . .less than 10,000 psi/sec
Ignition temperature−cloud . . . . .300°C and higher
Ignition temperature−layer . . . . .150°C and higher

This list points up the most significant difference between Class I gas or vapor hazards and Class II dust hazards. Though other characteristics are similar, the minimum ignition energy of even the more easily ignited industrial dusts is 20 times greater than that of typical Class I Group D materials.

It is possible to generalize about the explosion hazard of materials within some classes of dust on the basis of chemical composition. In the class of carbonaceous dusts, including carbons, charcoal, coal, coke, graphite, lignite, asphalt, and related materials, hazard is closely related to volatile content. If volatile content is below 8%, as it is in many carbons and charcoals, there may be a fire hazard, but there is essentially no dust explosion hazard. Lignite, pitch, and asphaltic materials with volatile content of 30−40%, on the other hand, present a severe dust explosion hazard.

Within the class of dusts frequently found in the plastics industry, explosion hazard and chemical structure are intimately related and inferences can be drawn on the basis of structural differences. For details see Bureau of Mines Report RI 5971.

The figures quoted above are typical of dry (less than 5% moisture) materials without appreciable inert material. Addition of moisture or inert material, in general, provides heat absorbing mass without increasing the amount of energy released. (Many metal dusts reacting with water and moisture may, on the contrary, increase explosion severity.) At a specific dust concentration, moderate amounts of moisture or inert material do not markedly change ignition energy, maximum pressure, or rate of pressure rise, but the effects increase rapidly as the amount of moisture or inert material approaches the value which quenches the explosion. Typically, the moisture level must be 15–50% of the dust concentration to prevent ignition by a strong inductive spark. The percentage of inert material, such as fuller's earth, required to prevent spark ignition is frequently as high as 90%. In general, the efficacy of inerting material is related to its heat capacity. However, the alkali salts are much more effective than their relative heat capacity would suggest. Minimum concentration for ignition increases linearly with either moisture or dry inert addition.

INFLUENCE OF SHAPE, SIZE, AND CONCENTRATION

As one would expect, the shape, size, and concentration of the suspended dust has a significant effect on ease of ignition and the properties of the explosion. Irregularly shaped particles produced by milling and grinding operations which have a high area-to-volume ratio are more easily ignited and represent a more severe explosion hazard than spherical particles produced by operations like spray drying.

Experimental data verify the almost obvious relationship between particle size and explosion hazard, because the finer the dust, the more homogeneous the cloud, and the greater the surface area for reaction.

The relationship between particle size and the important hazard parameters is summarized below. The conclusions are for a range of particle sizes of 0.001 in. to 0.012 in.

Ignition temperature . . . . . .Relatively independent of size
Maximum pressure (closed
   chamber) . . . . .Slight dependence
Minimum concentration   Below 0.003 in. little depend-
  (oz/ft^3) . . . .   ence
                          Above 0.003 in. inversely pro-
                           portional to size
Minimum ignition energy Inversely proportional to par-
Rate of pressure rise   ticle diameter.

Particle sizes larger than those for which conclusions are drawn above are not important in determining explosion hazard. It has been reported that 0.015 in. cornstarch or fuller's earth particles are the largest that affect the development of an explosion, and that the average cornstarch particle size of 0.028 in. is the largest that will ignite in air.

Metal dusts in particular may react quite differently if particle size is smaller than the above range. Very small particles, approximately 40×10^{-6} in. in diameter, will ignite solely because of exothermic reaction with oxygen; sometimes even in a layer.

Othmer and Schwab confirmed the relationships reported by the Bureau of Mines, and further emphasized that rate of pressure rise is determined by the amount of oxygen present. There is therefore an optimum surface area for the dust particles in a given chamber volume. As particle size increases, the concentration in weight per unit volume must thus increase. They also show that in a vented chamber the inverse dependence of rate of pressure rise on particle diameter causes the maximum pressure attained to increase as particle size is decreased. The effect is, of course, dependent on the amount of venting, but some venting will occur in almost every industrial situation.

In Chapters 3 and 4, it was shown that for spark ignition, the ignition energy of gases and vapors changed markedly with concentration, and there exists a well-defined, most easily ignited concentration. This is not true of dusts. Ignition energy drops from a relatively high value at the minimum concentration for ignition to the minimum value. Further increase in concentration does not materially change the energy requirement. Cloud ignition temperature also drops to a low value and remains essentially constant.

There are peaks in both the maximum rate of rise in pressure and the maximum pressure reached during an explosion. They peak at different concentrations, but both at concentrations 5—10 times stoichiometric. Excess dust does not act as an inerting material

Another distinctive feature of dust hazards is that there is no well-defined U.E.L. For practical purposes it does not exist.

CHEMICAL COMPOSITION OF THE SUSPENDING MEDIUM

The effect of reducing the oxygen content is similar to the effect of adding moisture or dry inert material. The explosion characteristics change slowly at first, and then very rapidly as the oxygen concentration approaches the limit value for the particular dust composition and geometry.

The diluent used to reduce oxygen content is effective in proportion to its molar heat capacity. Carbon dioxide is a more effective diluent than nitrogen. At high temperatures water vapor is as effective as carbon dioxide.

Argon and helium are preferable diluents for metal dusts. Many metals react with carbon dioxide or nitrogen. The hydrides of thorium, uranium, and zirconium, however, are preferably inerted with carbon dioxide.

Table 11-1 lists properties of some typical dust samples. The references listed at the end of this chapter include a wealth of other data; the table is merely illustrative of these. Sample-to-sample differences are large, even for the same material. It is important to note that the cloud ignition temperature determined by blowing a dust cloud against hot furnace walls is frequently several hundred degrees higher than the layer ignition temperature. The latter temperature is determined by raising the temperature of a dust layer in an oven. It is probably time-dependent for many materials. Dehydration and changes in composition occurring over long exposure to elevated temperatures below the reported layer ignition temperature will, in some cases at least, result in ignition at a lower temperature than that reported.

In Chapter 4 it was pointed out that reported ignition energy data for gases and vapors are conservatively biased because conditions in the laboratory are contrived to be more favorable to ignition than conditions to be expected in the field. Dust ignition data are also conservative for the same reason. Experimenters use well maintained electrode systems whose geometry is highly favorable to ignition, and use the most easily ignited concentration. In addition, the effects of particle size and moisture content also are weighted in favor of ignition. In Bureau of Mines work, particle size was 200 mesh or finer in almost all cases, and moisture content was reduced with few exceptions below 5% before testing. As noted earlier, minimum ignition energy is inversely related to particle diameter. In a real cloud it is unlikely that the dust particles would be as fine as through 200 mesh. Although larger particles will settle out, tending to leave only fine particles in suspension, the fine particles tend to agglomerate. Reduction of

TABLE 11-1. Explosion Characteristics of Typical Dusts

Type of dust	Ignition temp., °C		Ignition energy, mJ	L.E.L., oz/ft^3	Max. explosion pressure, psi	Max. rate, psi/sec
	Cloud	Layer				
Metal Powders (RI6516)						
Aluminum, atomized	650	760	50	0.045	73	20,000+
Iron, carbonyl	320	310	20	0.105	41	2,400
Magnesium, atomized	620	490	40	0.040	90	9,000
Manganese	460	240	305	0.125	48	2,800
Silicon		790	100	0.110	82	12,000
Tin	630	430	80	0.190	37	1,300
Titanium	330	510	25	0.045	70	5,500
Vanadium	500	490	60	0.220	48	600
Zinc	680	460	960	0.500	48	1,800
Dowmetal	430	480	80	0.020	86	10,000
Zirconium	20	190	15 max.	0.045	55	6,500
Plastics (RI5971)						
Casein	520	—	60	0.045	73	1,000
Cellulose Acetates	470	400	25	0.045	135	6,000
Methyl methacrylate	440	—	15	0.020	101	1,800
Phenolic resin	580	—	10	0.025	89	8,500
Polyethylene resin	450	—	80	0.025	83	2,500
Polystyrene	490	—	120	0.020	62	1,500
Shellac, rosin, gum	400	—	10	0.020	73	3,600
Synthetic rubber, hard	320	—	30	0.030	93	3,100
Urea molding compound	460	—	80	0.085	89	3,600
Vinyl butyral resin	390	—	10	0.020	84	2,000
Agricultural Products (RI5753)						
Alfalfa	470	220	370	0.160	76	800
Cocoa	510	200	100	0.045	68	1,400
Coffee	720	270	160	0.085	38	150
Cornstarch	380	330	40	0.055	58	2,200
Cotton linters	520	—	1,920	0.500	44	400
Egg whites	610	—	640	0.140	58	500
Garlic	360	—	240	0.100	57	1,300
Milk, skim	490	200	50	0.050	95	2,300
Nut shells, pecan	440	210	50	0.030	112	3,500
Pectin	410	200	35	0.075	132	7,000
Rice	440	240	50	0.050	105	2,700
Sugar	370	400	30	0.045	109	5,000
Wheat Flour	440	440	60	0.050	97	2,800

moisture content of course reduces the energy required to evaporate the moisture during ignition.

DISTINGUISHING FEATURES OF DUST HAZARDS

Though the small-scale ignition processes of dust explosions are not greatly different from those of gas and vapor explosions, the gross nature of dust hazards is sufficiently different from gas and vapor hazards to require different techniques of hazard reduction. Dust hazards are cumulative, whereas gas or vapor hazards are dispersive. If process equipment releases a combustible vapor or gas the hazard is usually only transient. Even heavier-than-air vapors trapped in low spots are eventually dispersed or diffused. Should a second release of combustible material occur the effects are usually independent of the first release. Dust hazards, on the other hand, accumulate. Dust settles out of the air eventually and is stored for future combustion on beams, windowsills, and equipment. Fortunately, the dust hazard is visible and obvious from the moment the hazard first exists. The L.E.L. of wheat flour, 0.05 oz/ft^3, is equivalent to about one-half teaspoon per cubic foot, not an unnoticeable concentration by any means. Before the concentration reaches the L.E.L., visibility is reduced to a few feet and breathing is difficult.

Although air currents can carry a gas or vapor hazard to a great distance from the source of combustible material, primary dust hazards exist mostly at processing machinery where air currents keep dust continuously in suspension, or the processing equipment continuously feeds more dust into the air to replace that which has settled. A true Division 1 dust area is in most cases quite limited. However, because of the conservative nature of dust hazards, a very real hazard may exist in a large area surrounding a Division 1 area.

If a small cloud of gas or vapor ignites, the entire supply of combustible material is burned in a single explosion. The combustion wave does not travel farther than the extent of the combustible gas or vapor. On the other hand, if a small cloud of dust ignites, the resulting puff, harmless in itself, and causing no damage, may dislodge additional dust from nearby equipment. This new and larger cloud ignites, causes a larger blast, shakes more dust into the atmosphere, and the resulting series of explosions may demolish a structure, though the initiating explosion was harmless by itself. The only sure means of stopping multiple explosions of this sort is good housekeeping practice in buildings of design such as to discourage the accumulation of dust layers.

Othmer and Schwab note that multiple explosions of a different variety occur, and that these are the reason why industrial dust explosion damage is often puzzling: windows, doors, and walls collapse inwardly. They state that after the first puff has shaken down a large dust cloud which ignites, the resulting explosion consumes all of the oxygen, but not all of the dust. After this explosion air rushes into the building, causing inward collapse of walls, and the remaining unburned dust ignites to cause another explosion. This process may repeat itself.

The conservative nature of the dust hazard also leads to another problem not found in Class I locations, the accumulation of thermally insulating blankets of dust on equipment. Equipment must not only have surface temperatures well below the layer ignition temperature of the dust, but the equipment must maintain these low temperatures even when a dust layer accumulates and interferes with conduction of heat away from the equipment.

AREA CLASSIFICATION

In practice, classification of Class II and Class III hazardous locations is in the majority of cases less systematic even than classification of Class I locations. There is a greater tendency to classify all areas Division 1, or at least to specify equipment suitable for Division 1 locations even in Division 2 or nonhazardous locations.

One company, however, has used sampling instruments to determine that even in those Class II locations where dust clouds are heaviest the concentrations are well below the L.E.L. reported by the Bureau of Mines. Insurance underwriters have, on the basis of the evidence, approved installation of Division 2 equipment.

One criterion for determining whether a location is Division 1 is the presence of a cloud of dust of greater than minimum concentration, regularly, frequently, or intermittently. In order for an explosion to occur dust must be in suspension. If there is a blanket but no cloud there can be ignition and fire, but no immediate explosion. There can be explosion only if thermal turbulence from the fire causes dust to become suspended.

A location will also be Division 1 if the dust is electrically conductive or if electrical failure and dust release are caused by the same occurrence. A location may therefore be considered to be a Division 2 location if process equipment failure may loose a dust cloud of explosive concentration; or if the dust layer is in a location where it may be ignited by faulty equipment and there is sufficient volume to ignite.

If equipment with a 55°C temperature rise over 40°C ambient is used, and the color of the equipment can be seen through the dust layer, the area is almost certainly nonhazardous. There is no cloud. The layer is not thick enough to seriously retard heat dissipation and it is not thick enough to propagate a flame. Unfortunately, it is not possible to say how much thicker the layer must be to warrant a Division 2 classification.

MEANS OF REDUCING DUST HAZARD

Primary dust hazards tend to eliminate themselves because dust settles out of the air. The extent of the hazard can therefore best be localized to essential processing equipment by good house-keeping. In other respects the philosophy of protection and hazard reduction is the same as that outlined in Chapter 5 for gases and vapors. However, the specific methods used for reducing gas and vapor hazards are not necessarily applicable to dust hazards.

Explosion-proof or flameproof enclosures are not necessarily applicable to dust hazards. Gaps which are quite permissible in gas or vapor hazards may permit the entry of dust into the equipment. Enclosures approved for Class I may also be approved for Class II and Class III hazards, but such dual rating is not automatic.

Enclosures suitable for Class II hazards are "dust-ignition-proof" enclosures, specified by the NEC to be used in Division 1 locations for switches, circuit breakers, and similar equipment; and "tight metal enclosures... designed to minimize the entrance of dust," specified for Division 2 locations or for resistors or nonswitching applications in Division 1.

The latter enclosure need have only tight fitting or telescoping covers and no openings through which, after installation, sparks or burning material might escape, or through which exterior accumulations of dust might be ignited. They are used for both Division 1 and Division 2 installations in Class III locations. Dust-ignition-proof enclosures are designed to exclude dust. They must be of substantial construction; metal-to-metal joints are preferred, at least $\frac{3}{16}$ in. wide. However, gaskets may be used if they are mechanically affixed. Glued gaskets are not acceptable; rubber gaskets are not acceptable. In general, only certain inorganic gasketing compounds may be used.

Dust-ignition-proof enclosures are tested in a chamber full of swirling dust, with intermittent loading of the equipment inside the enclosure so that cycling temperature will increase the likelihood that the enclosure will breathe in dust. Equipment is examined to determine whether dust has entered. There must not be sufficient dust present to suggest that after several years' operation in a dusty atmosphere there could accumulate enough material to interfere with operation or create a material fire or explosion hazard. There must, of course, be no ignition. There shall be no charring of a blanket of dust on the surface of the enclosure. Surface temperatures are limited to 165°C maximum, or 120°C maximum, if the device, such as a motor or transformer, may be overloaded. All enclosures for conductive dusts must be specifically approved.

The application of sealing and potting procedures for equipment to be used in dust hazards is reasonable and the requirements are essentially the same as those for gas or vapors. Oil immersion per se would not seem to be a useful technique for dust hazards unless the enclosure were also dust-tight, which would be sufficient protection. Oil-immersed equipment is used, however, because of increased reliability of the switchgear, not for increased safety.

In mining practice inert dusts (rock) are added to combustible dusts to decrease ignitability. This technique cannot be widely applied. Addition of inert material to compose 90% of the mixture with agricultural dusts is required to entirely prevent ignition. As a practical matter, therefore, the technique is not applicable to foodstuffs. Gas inerting, however, can be applied to foodstuffs and other material where solid inerting is not permissible.

The application of intrinsically safe and nonincendive equipment to dust hazards is obvious, practical, and relatively easy compared to most gas and vapor applications, because the most easily ignited dusts have minimum ignition energies of approximately 10 mJ.

A recommended practice is now being prepared by Subcommittee B of ISA 8D-RP12. It seems to the author unlikely that the Recommended Practice for dusts will differ in philosophy from that for gases and vapors. It is almost certain that any device which is intrinsically safe for pentane group materials will be intrinsically safe for dusts, except that protection against hot wire or hot surface ignition may require different practice in Class II locations.

Purging is used at the present time as a means of improving reliability of switching and motor control circuits. Positive pressure excludes dust and prevents buildup of insulating dust layers on contacts. Arguments have been advanced that purging may not be applicable to Class II and III hazards because the purge air might stir up settled dust and increase hazard. Others feel that purging systems similar if not identical to those described in ISA RP12.4 will be utilized in other than Class I locations. They minimize the danger of stirring up any dust layer. In support of this view is the fact that in order to entrain settled dust air velocity must reach 6000–8000 ft/min. Even to convey already suspended dust requires velocities of 2000 ft/min. Purge pressures of a few inches of water and the restricted flow in a practical purge system make entrainment unlikely.

REFERENCES

1. Underwriters' Laboratories, Inc., Standards for Safety No. 698, "Industrial Control Equipment for Use in Hazardous Locations," 6th Edition, December, 1949.
2. National Electrical Code, Articles 502–503.
3. Jacobson, Nagy, Cooper, and Ball, "Explosibility of Agricultural Dusts," RI 5753, U.S. Bureau of Mines, Pittsburgh.
4. Riddlestone, H. G., and R. W. Coram, "Dust-Tight Enclosures for Electrical Apparatus: Examination of a Proposed Method of Test: D/T118," British Electrical and Allied Industries Research Association, 1960.
5. Marks, Lionel S., Mechanical Engineers Handbook, pp. 795–800, 5th Edition, 1951.
6. Jacobson, Nagy, and Cooper, "Explosibility of Dusts Used in the Plastics Industry," Bureau of Mines, RI 5971, 1962.
7. Hartmann, Cooper, Jacobson, "Recent Studies on the Explosibility of Cornstarch," Bureau of Mines, RI 4725, 1950.
8. Dorsett, Jacobson, Nagy, and Williams, "Laboratory Equipment and Test Procedures for Evaluating Explosibility of Dusts," Bureau of Mines, RI 5624, 1960.
9. Jacobson, Cooper, and Nagy, "Explosibility of Metal Powders," Bureau of Mines, RI 6516, 1964.
10. Nagy, Dorsett, Jacobson, "Preventing Ignition of Dust Dispersions by Inerting," Bureau of Mines, RI 6543, 1964.
11. Nagy, Cooper, Stupar, "Pressure Development in Laboratory Dust Explosion," Bureau of Mines, RI 6561, 1964.

Chapter 12
What Lies Ahead?

In the past decade acceptance of the principle of intrinsic safety has increased exponentially. During the next decade the problems of electrical safety will more and more be accepted as engineering problems amenable to solution by rational analysis and experiment. Electrically ignited explosions will be considered on the basis of technical factors, rather than on emotional ones.

The concepts needed for adequate and economical electrical safety are available. The most essential data and guides for applying these concepts are available. However, there are still many problem areas, where for lack of adequate understanding of ignition mechanisms judgment must be exercised. Judgment is not inherently undesirable, but judgment in lieu of knowledge usually costs money.

Many contributions to our knowledge of ignition mechanisms are needed. More experimental data and better theories which correlate the empirical data are required. Some of the subjects needing further study are noted below. It is hoped that by describing these subjects, readers of this book will be led to encourage technical work in these areas, so that more and more of the characteristics of devices necessary to safety can be quantified and codified.

Discharge of RC Circuits. It was pointed out in Chapter 4 that the amount of effort required to obtain ignition data has caused most experimenters to limit their work to a few simple cases. A case of considerable practical importance which has not been thoroughly explored either experimentally or theoretically is the effect of series resistance on the amount of energy required for ignition by discharging capacitors in low-voltage circuits. It is known that relatively few ohms can markedly increase the amount of energy required. However, theory and experimental data are still inadequate for design of an optimum circuit. Therefore, resistors must be sized on the assumption that the capacitor is an infinite source. This frequently is ultraconservative and uneconomic.

Effects of Electrode Geometry. Every experimenter determines a new set of ignition energy data. If he is attempting to develop test equipment to produce ignition at some desired level, he modifies contact geometry or speed to make his apparatus produce ignition at that energy level. He can predict direction of change but not magnitude. It is likely that the energy which could be dissipated in arcing contacts could be increased to amazingly high values if the contacts themselves were designed to quench efficiently. Here is a challenging area for theoretical and experimental work.

Ignition Theory. A quantitative theory of ignition to supplant qualitative explanations is needed in order to relate data from different sources and correlate ignition by different mechanisms.

Hot-Wire Ignition. There are many unanswered questions about hot-wire ignition. Little work has been done with gases and vapors other than methane and hydrogen. Although hot-wire ignition is not of critical concern to the instrument industry, a better understanding of the facts and theory of hot-wire ignition would certainly be a contribution to the art.

Inductors with Dissipative Cores. There is a fertile field of great practical importance in the development of design equations for iron or ferrite cored devices. Work is needed to define those parameters which make the discharge of stored energy inefficient and to quantify them for design purposes. Other work is needed to define those situations where material properties and volume effectively limit the amount of stored energy in the inductor.

Measurement of Dust Concentration. Available instruments for measuring concentration in a dust cloud are not entirely satisfactory because the sampling time is considerably longer than the time required for an explosion to develop. Infrequent short-duration high-concentration clouds would not be indicated by such devices. A one-millisecond rise-time instrument inexpensive enough for plant survey work is required.

Time—Temperature Effects in Layer Ignition. Chemical changes and dehydration of dusts maintained at temperatures below the initial layer ignition temperature eventually causes the layer ignition temperature to decrease. More investigation of these effects is required. In some cases, the 160°C U.L. surface temperature limit for equipment not subject to overloads is already too high.

Criteria for Conductive Dusts. Metal and carbonaceous dusts pose a peculiar problem because they are electrically conductive. Where they exist, the location is classified Division 1. Research is needed to establish how conductive a dust must be to pose a real hazard.

Index